Auburn Public Library

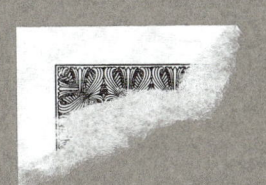

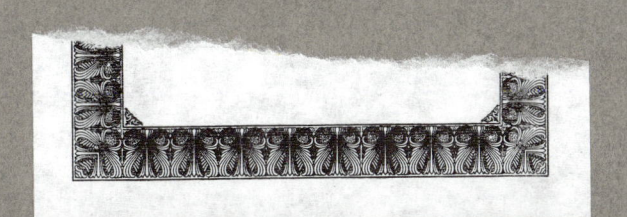

111699

362.196 KAR / Body & Soul ANONF

Y0-ADZ-291

MAY 31 '05	DATE DUE	
OCT 18 '06		

Body & Soul

Body &

THE COURAGE
OF BREAST CAN

by Jean

EMMIS ⓔ BOOKS

& Soul

AND BEAUTY
CER SURVIVORS

Karotkin

CINCINNATI, OHIO

Copyright 2004 by Jean Karotkin

All rights reserved. No portion of this book may be reproduced in any fashion, print, facsimile, or electronic, or by any other method yet to be developed, without express permission of the copyright holder.

For further information, contact the publisher at

emmis
books

Emmis Books
1700 Madison Road
Cincinnati, OH 45206

www.emmisbooks.com

ISBN 1-57860-152-5

Library of Congress Cataloging-in-Publication Data

Karotkin, Jean, 1949-
  Body & soul : the courage and beauty of breast cancer survivors / by Jean Karotkin.
    p. cm.
  ISBN 1-57860-152-5
  1. Breast—Cancer—Patients—Portraits. I. Title: Body and soul. II. Title.
  RC280.B8K353 2004
  362.196'99449'00922—dc22
                    2004053229

Book design by DJ Stout and Erin Mayes, Pentagram Design Inc.
Edited by Jessica Yerega
Printed in Mexico by RR Donnelley

For my daughter,
Suzanne

Acknowledgements

Since the conception of this project in 1995, I have traveled an amazing road. I have bonded and connected with so many incredible women and men who have helped me to bring this dream to fruition.

Richard Abdo, who implemented the foundation and tools to change my life positively—mentally and physically—after breast cancer.

To my parents, all my love.

Michael R. Levy, my brother and publisher of *Texas Monthly*. Because of his understanding of my vision of the project from the beginning, his numerous introductions were incredibly beneficial.

Rebecca Cohen, my friend and mother of my nieces, who believed from the beginning that through my eyes I could make this happen. Her gifted talent as a writer helped me numerous times with letters of introduction. Her gentle manner and thoughtful choice of words could always be counted on to boost my confidence at any given moment.

Tobin Levy, Rachel Goldberg, and Mara Levy for their devotion, encouragement, and numerous suggestions.

DJ Stout with Pentagram Design Inc., who supported my work from the beginning and whose genius as a designer brought this book to life.

Erin Mayes with Pentagram Design Inc. for being a part of the design team.

David Rucker and Nikki Mason, with The Mark, whose amazing talent for processing and printing black-and-white film have truly been beneficial in bringing my images to the pages here.

Beca Sticher for her amazing craft of eliminating those imperfections to polish the finished images.

Cathy Casey, senior editor of *Texas Monthly*, who believed in the project and introduced me to Emmis Books publisher Richard Hunt, to whom I owe a debt of gratitude for making my dream come true in publishing the book.

Jessica Yerega, my editor at Emmis Books, for her assistance in helping me bring to life the stories behind the images.

The team at Emmis Books for assisting Richard and Jessica in bringing this book to fruition.

Rick Eilers, my mentor and first photography teacher.

Travis Ueoka, Karen Davenport, and Julia Hunt, my teachers and colleagues at Brookhaven Community College.

Dr. George Peters, my champion and saint of breast cancer surgeons at Southwestern Medical of Dallas.

Lynn Sugarman, who gave me the opportunity to use her amazing studio to photograph my first image.

Lisa Tench Bearden of Sunwest Publishing Inc., who gave me continued support for the images and the cause.

Steve Stuyke, vice president of public affairs at MD Anderson Cancer Center, and Jo Ann Ward, executive director of public education at MD Anderson, who both graciously volunteered their support and direction.

Barbara Hurwitz, a member of MD Anderson's board of visitors, for her efforts and support in hosting an exhibit of my images at the Saks/MD Anderson Cancer Center gala.

Susan Rafte, co-founder of the Pink Ribbon Project in Houston, for her enthusiastic support and participation with the project, and for allowing my work to be a part of her Pink Ribbon Gala.

Rebecca Myers, for writing a wonderful article for the American Cancer Society's newsletter, and for her continued support.

Jane Parker and Linda Conner, with the Susan G. Komen affiliate in Houston, who exhibited my images.

Becky Delaune, with the Susan G. Komen affiliate in Fort Worth, for displaying the images during a benefit at the Fort Worth Modern Museum.

Judy Rosenblum and John Broude, for being my best cheerleaders and assisting me in every way imaginable.

Edna and Drew Robins, Leslie Field, Claire and Doug Ankenman, Cindy and Ronny Bass, Bonnie Likeover, Eva Wolski and Marc Grossberg, and Joy and Brent Ford, my dear friends in Houston who opened so many doors for me, helping me to meet these wonderful women to photograph, assisting me with finding shooting locations, and making introductions to promote the project for exhibition.

Jean Caslin, director of the Houston Center for Photography, for the gift of exhibiting my work and understanding the importance of educating the community about breast cancer.

Marlene Kahan, executive director of the American Society of Magazine Editors, who made numerous phone calls to magazines on my behalf.

Tracey Smith, with NBC's *Today*, and Stephanie Saft, former producer of the *Today* show, who were responsible for making possible the amazing experience of showing my images nationally and being interviewed by Ann Curry.

Bobbi Queen, associate fashion editor of *W* magazine, who came forth with amazing women to meet and photograph in New York.

The former staff of *Rosie Magazine* for giving me the opportunity to photograph and meet six amazing women from different parts of the country.

Beatris Terrazas, staff writer for the "Living" section of the *Dallas Morning News*, for her coverage of the project.

The staff of *O, the Oprah Magazine* for publishing a selection of my images for a related story on breast cancer survivors.

Louise Snyder in Gross Point, Michigan, for her efforts to introduce me to some amazing women in her area to photograph and for being my guardian during my visit.

Roxanne Isbey, my longtime friend in New York, who connected me with other women in the city to photograph for the book. I thank you for securing me free room and board as well as great photo assistants during my photo shoots.

Cindy Stanley, Benjamin Sanderford, Tina and Dolph Simon, Betty and Steve Silverman, and Debbie Tolson, whose friendships have been so important.

To all of the women who allowed me to photograph them and share their stories, I thank you from the bottom of my heart. This dream never would have come true without you. I am truly blessed.

Introduction

Ten years ago, I picked up the *New York Times* magazine to find a partially disrobed, disarmingly beautiful woman on the cover. A mastectomy scar raked across her otherwise perfect torso. Her face radiated self-confidence. As I stared at the image, I felt as if someone had inched open a door that I never knew existed. That photograph conveyed what a sensitive spouse or more self-assured mother than my own should have made clear after my own mastectomy several years before: While cancer may claim a breast or shorten the years of a woman's life, it does not have the authority to compromise her beauty or to dilute the accomplishments that precede or follow treatment.

Under the spell of that photo I envisioned compiling an entire book filled with portraits of breast cancer survivors. I would find seasoned photographers to capture the femininity and sexuality of these women, to portray their grit and determination. Together we would assemble an inspiring, powerful portfolio that would not only accrue to women who had been diagnosed with cancer, but also would allow the subjects themselves to fully appreciate their own beauty and strength. Best of all, the project would provide a life-affirming role model for my daughter, who was burdened by our family's history of the disease. Three generations—her great-grandmother, her grandmother, and myself—have suffered with breast cancer. And low self-esteem also seemed to run in the family, at least where my mother and I were concerned. I was already planning to quietly shepherd the book into being, then relinquish control to others. I could not imagine traveling around the country by myself to talk with or to photograph strangers. The lost and lonely adolescent I had been—whose peers made fun of the back brace she wore to correct scoliosis—was still very much in control of my self-image. A failed marriage had left me stranded in a sea of self-doubt.

For two frustrating years I struggled in vain to find partners who would help me see the project to completion. To make matters worse, I broke my hip in a fall and spent several months recovering. It was only then, with the help of friends, that I began to hobble toward the realization that only I could make my dream come true. "Take the pictures yourself," urged my sister-in-law Becky, an arts writer who knew that I had studied photography as a hobby. I was terrified and intrigued at the prospect. Richard, my nutritionist, propped me up physically and emotionally. Lynn, a photographer friend who came to visit me at home while I was recovering from my fall, offered to let me use her studio and to help me set up my shoots for the first few sessions. Dana Ravel, still bald after a recent bout of stem cell therapy, agreed to be my first subject, despite being skeptical about the notion of wrapping herself in a towel for the camera. The feisty former art dealer refused to don the boxing gloves I wanted her to wear until I had only two rolls of film left. "Give me those things," she finally said, and then she assumed the position that I had envisioned so clearly—dukes up! With that first photograph, my journey began.

There were, of course, stumbling blocks along the way. Many of the women I approached were not comfortable in front of the camera and were unwilling to pose for me. Occasionally husbands advised their spouses against stepping into the spotlight. Others agreed to pose and then changed their minds at the last minute after I'd traveled halfway across the country to see them. But the ones with whom I've laughed and cried, the ones whose portraits appear in this book, have left me feeling incredibly proud to be a woman. I am in awe of every single one of them. Photographic sessions I'd arranged with a stranger frequently ended hours after they'd begun with a hug from a newly made friend.

My own experience with breast cancer pales in comparison to the ordeals endured by most of the women depicted here. I was one of the "lucky" ones for whom surgery—a simple mastectomy and subsequent reconstruction—was sufficient, without chemotherapy or radiation. And yet every annual checkup summons old fears. Sadly, a few of the women whose photographs appear on these pages, including that wonderful woman wearing the boxing gloves, have died. I take comfort in knowing that Dana lived each day with great vigor and joy, but I miss her still. Others will remain in treatment for years. "Cancer is always going to be in my life whether or not there's a reoccurrence. I have to learn how to walk with it," writes Oni Faida Lampley, whose photograph appears on page 30. Her words ring true. But does that walk with illness suggest that those who have cancer must surrender their autonomy, sexuality, creativity, or delight in life's pleasures? I think not. Gaze into the eyes of the women on the following pages. Take note of the sexy curves, elegant demeanors, dreamy expressions, and playful poses. They are aglow with life, despite or perhaps even because of their experience with breast cancer.

There are many choices to be made when a woman learns she has breast cancer. Most have to do with finding the best medical caregivers, agreeing on the most appropriate mode of treatment, and finding ways to continue to work and to care for family members. But there are other challenges as well, including learning to retain a sense of humor the way Liz Carpenter was able to do; defining oneself by life rather than illness like Gloria Stuart proposes; and relying on the support of partners and friends, as so many of the woman portrayed in this book have done, without losing a sense of self. It is my hope that "meeting" the women on these pages will help other breast cancer patients find an optimistic stance as they heal both body and soul. Just as I was inspired by that photograph ten years ago, I pray that others will be empowered to find the courage to open doors and to create a new and perhaps even better life after breast cancer, regardless of the odds or the outcome. It is my profound hope that these photos reveal to all the beauty, power, and life-affirming spirit that I saw through the camera's lens. I offer special thanks to the women whose pictures grace these pages for sharing my journey and for setting a fine example for me and for all of our daughters and sons, partners and friends.

Jerri

In 1999, the world watched as Jerri Nielsen, the only physician at an isolated South Pole research station, diagnosed and then directed her own breast cancer operation. Since leaving the Pole station in October of that year, she has lived by the ocean. In her book, *Ice Bound*, she writes, "There are times when the ocean is calm and flat as glass, and the horizon is empty for miles in every direction. Those are the times I feel at home again, and remember Antarctica."

Today, Jerri is living the dream of her life. She travels the world as a public speaker. She has a profound effect on women who are afraid. Her talks, and her book, instill courage. She says the friendships she has developed with other women through her travels have been her greatest gift. "I truly understand how necessary women are to society today. Women are such a great support to each other."

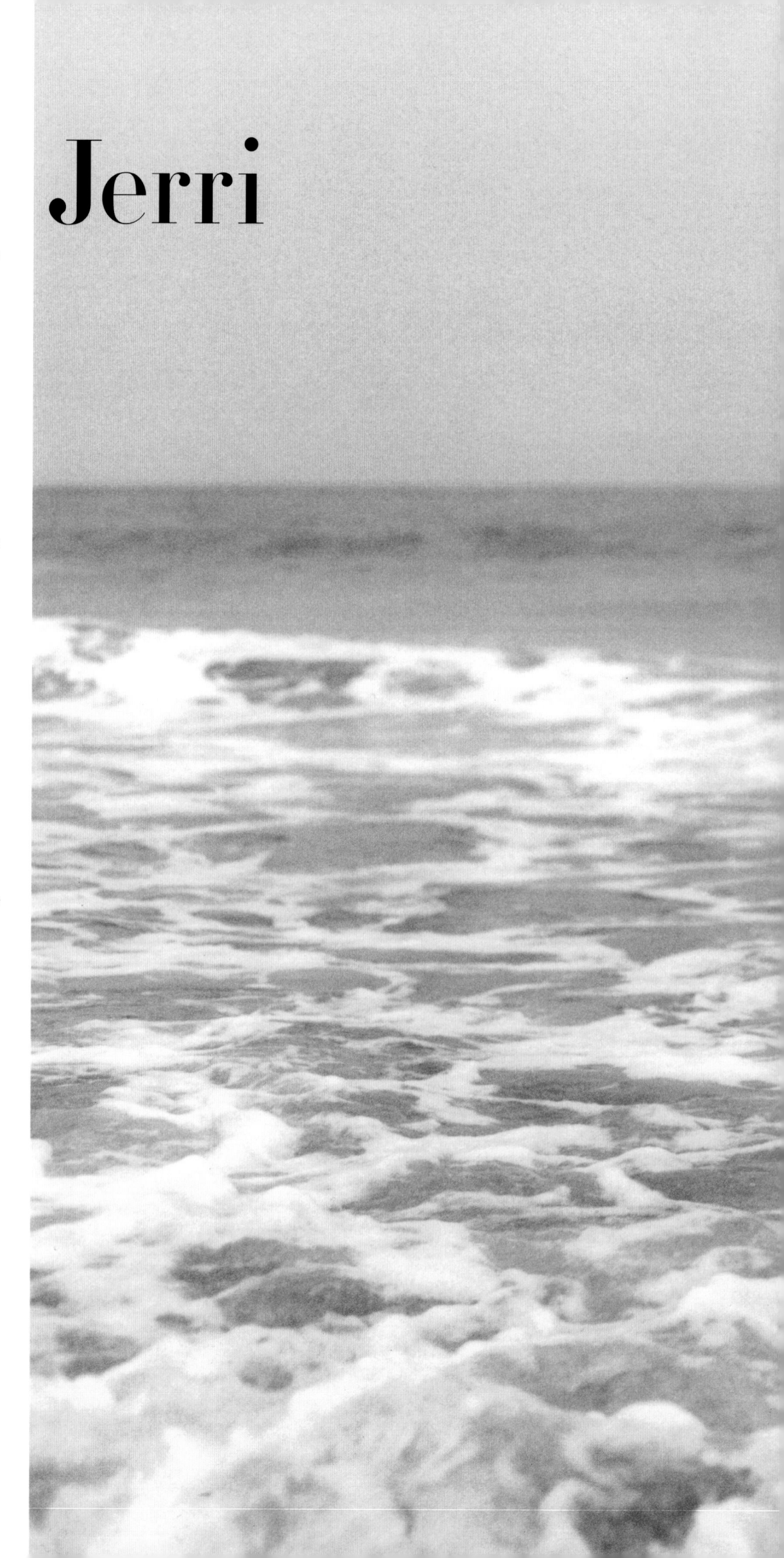

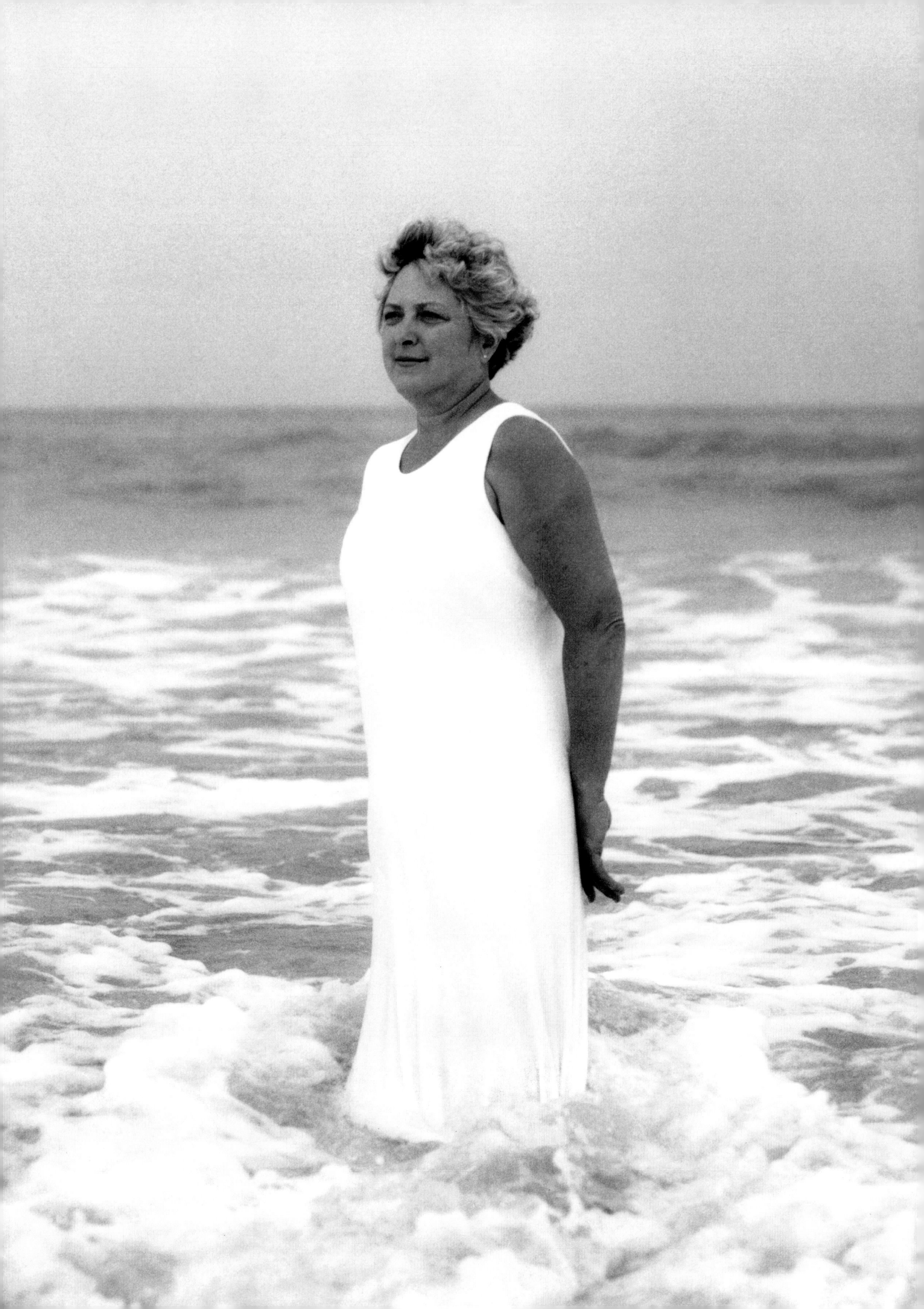

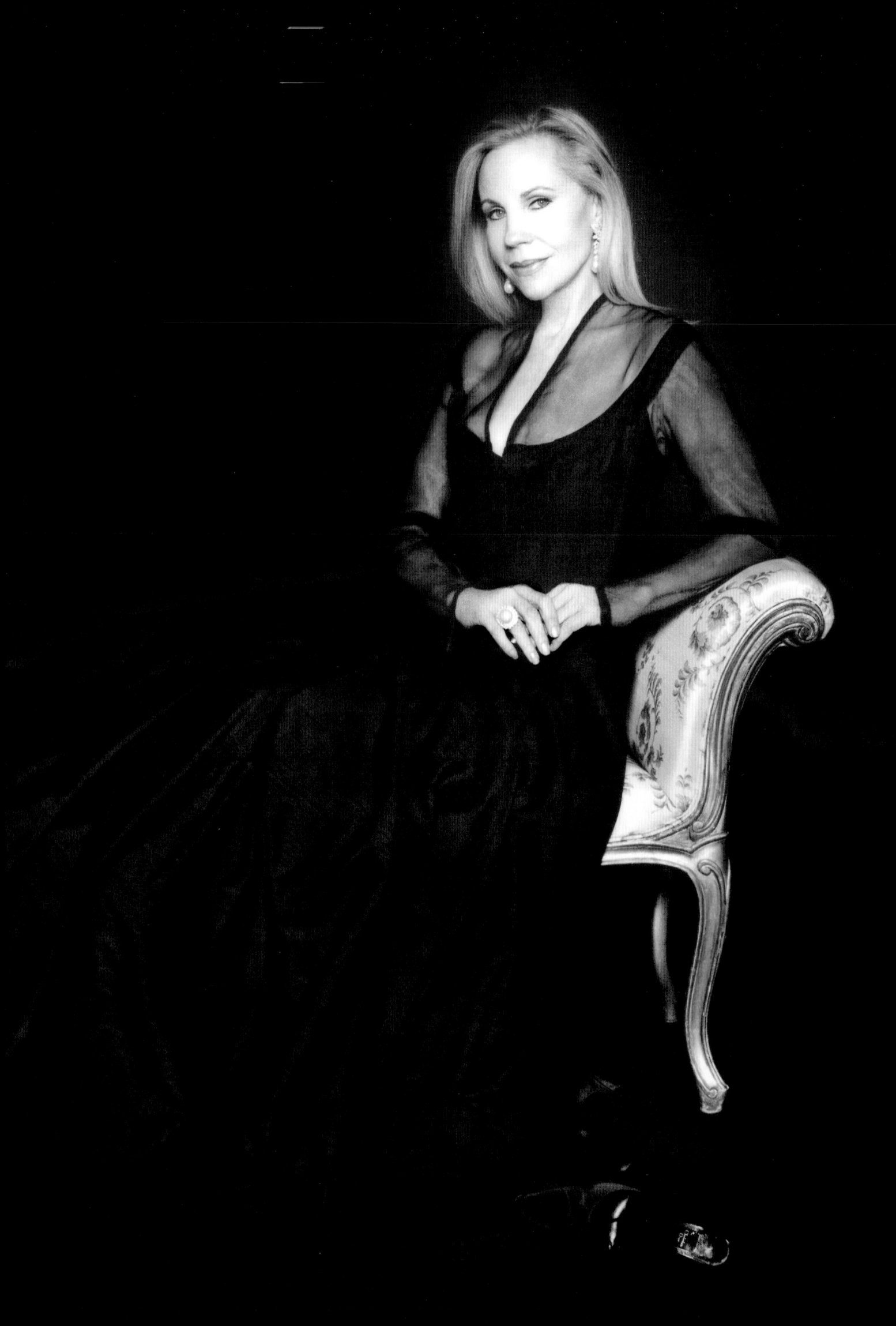

Carolyn

Carolyn Farb is notorious both in her hometown of Houston and across the country for her lifelong devotion to fundraising. She has raised more than thirty million dollars for a wide variety of charities and organizations in need. She identifies herself as a dreamer, a trailblazer, and a gifted communicator. "My work is my art," she says.

Carolyn's experience with breast cancer nine years ago didn't slow her down. "Before cancer, I felt invincible. In a moment, life changes. Cancer takes on a surreal experience. My days are filled with what matters and reaching for the stars."

Leah

Leah Garmon was a success in many areas of her life. She was a devoted wife and mother of three children, and she enjoyed a career as a wardrobe consultant for twenty-five years. She also was a member of her church's benevolence committee, and was committed to sharing her faith and hope, helping those less fortunate, mentoring young women, and visiting others who were fighting cancer.

When Leah was diagnosed with breast cancer, her drive for success and her faith became even more valuable to her. "See your beauty through God's eyes," she said. *Leah died in August 2002 at the age of forty-nine.*

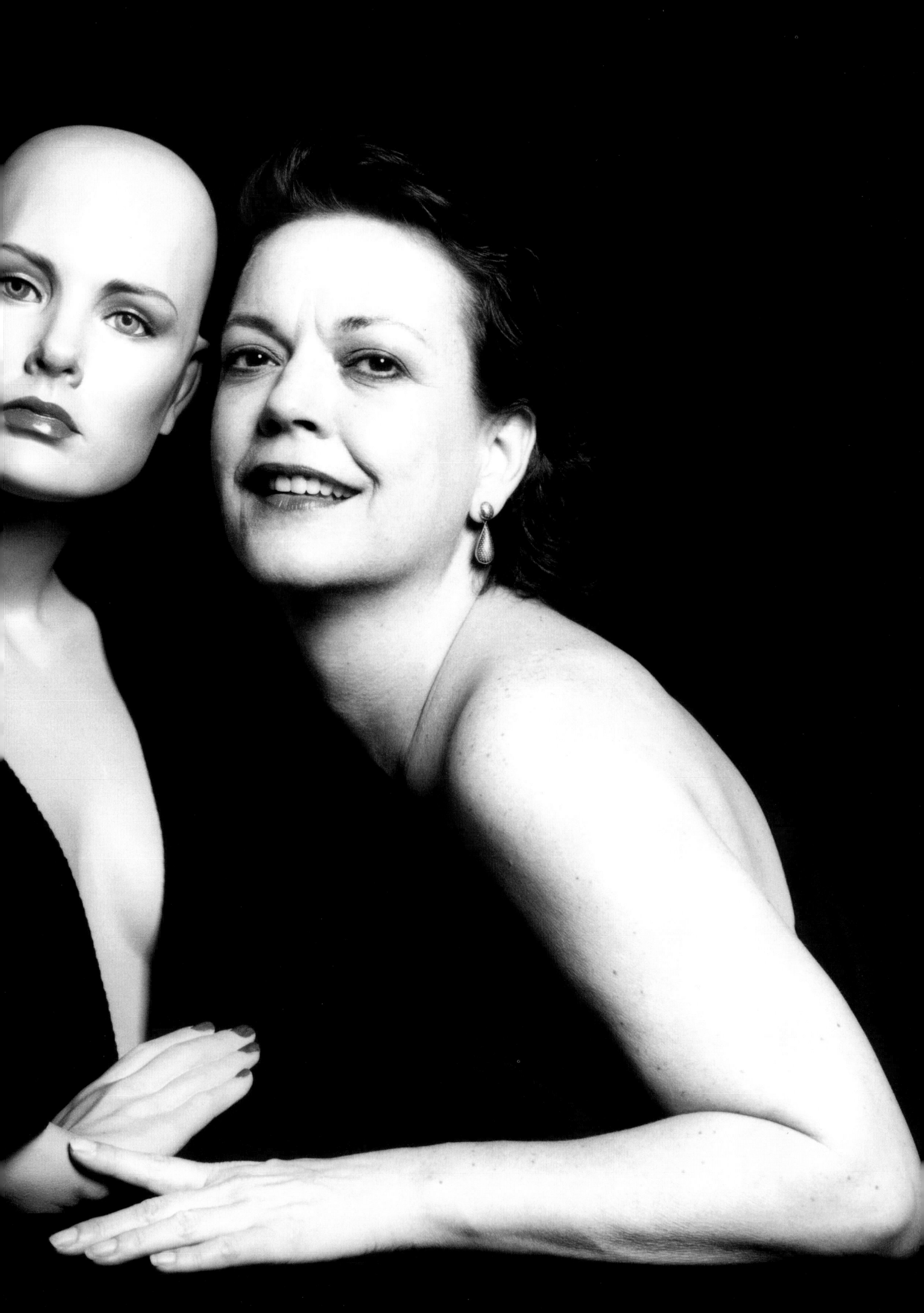

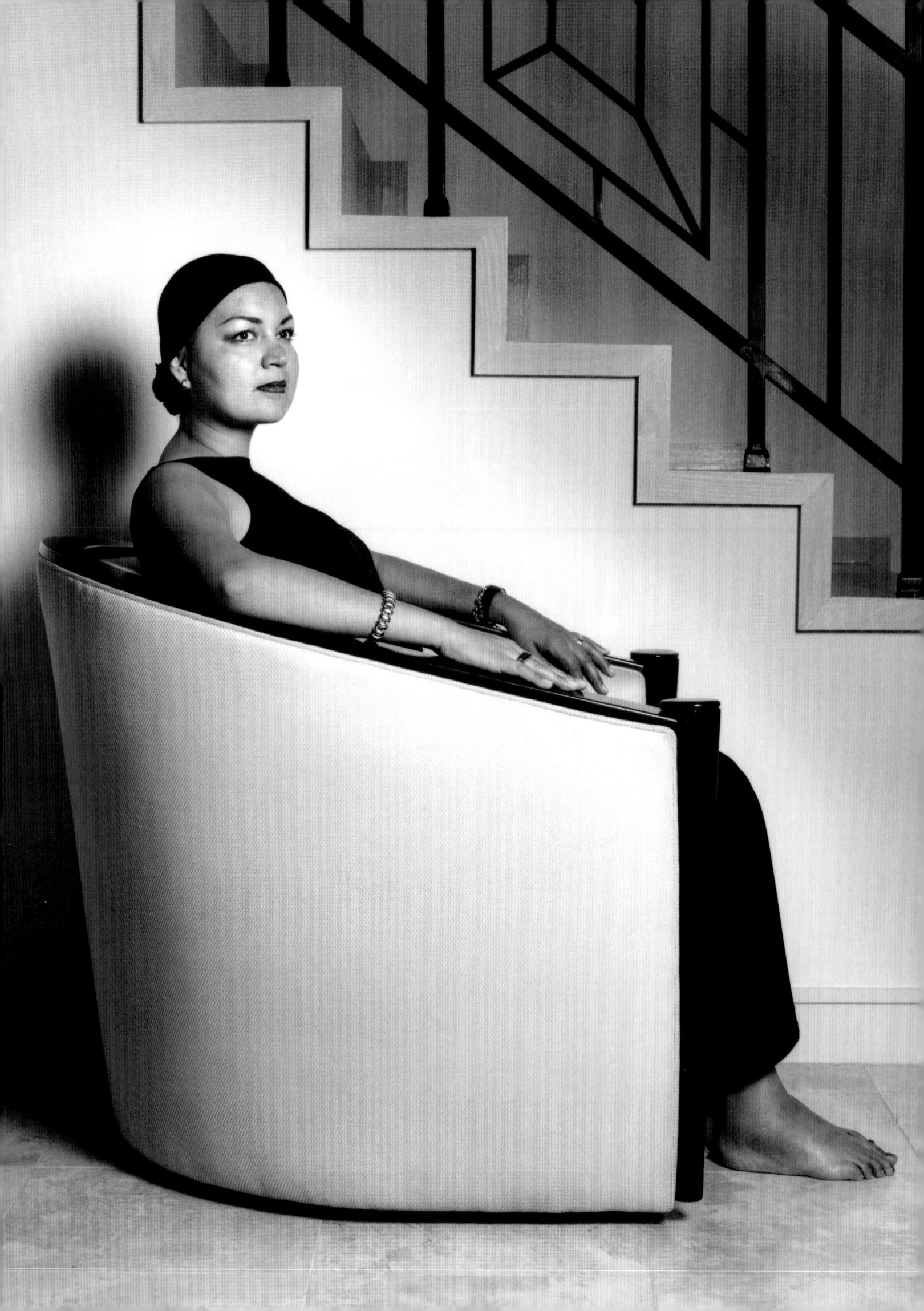

Martha

A native of Mexico, Martha Carrillo was only fifteen when her mother died tragically and unexpectedly. Years later, Martha was living a successful life in the Mexican city of Celaya as a mother, wife, and architect when she was diagnosed with breast cancer. She says that although she found her diagnosis frightening, she knew that her mom was her guardian angel.

With her region offering substandard health care to that available in the United States, she was forced to make difficult decisions regarding the enormous expenses associated with her treatment. She finally decided to travel to Houston, Texas, for her medical care—even though she had no idea how she would afford the $11,000 each one would cost. But miraculously, she always seemed to find a way to pay her medical bills—and Martha says she took it as a sign that her mom was taking care of her from above.

Susan

Susan Rafte and her sister founded the Pink Ribbon Project in Houston in 1995. The project is the first dance initiative founded solely for the purpose of increasing breast cancer awareness and raising money to help fight the disease. DanceCare, an emergency breast cancer fund for dancers, grew out of the Pink Ribbon Project's New York City office.

Susan says cancer had a strong impact on her life because she was diagnosed at age thirty-three, around the time her first child was born. She now considers her experience with the disease part of her identity.

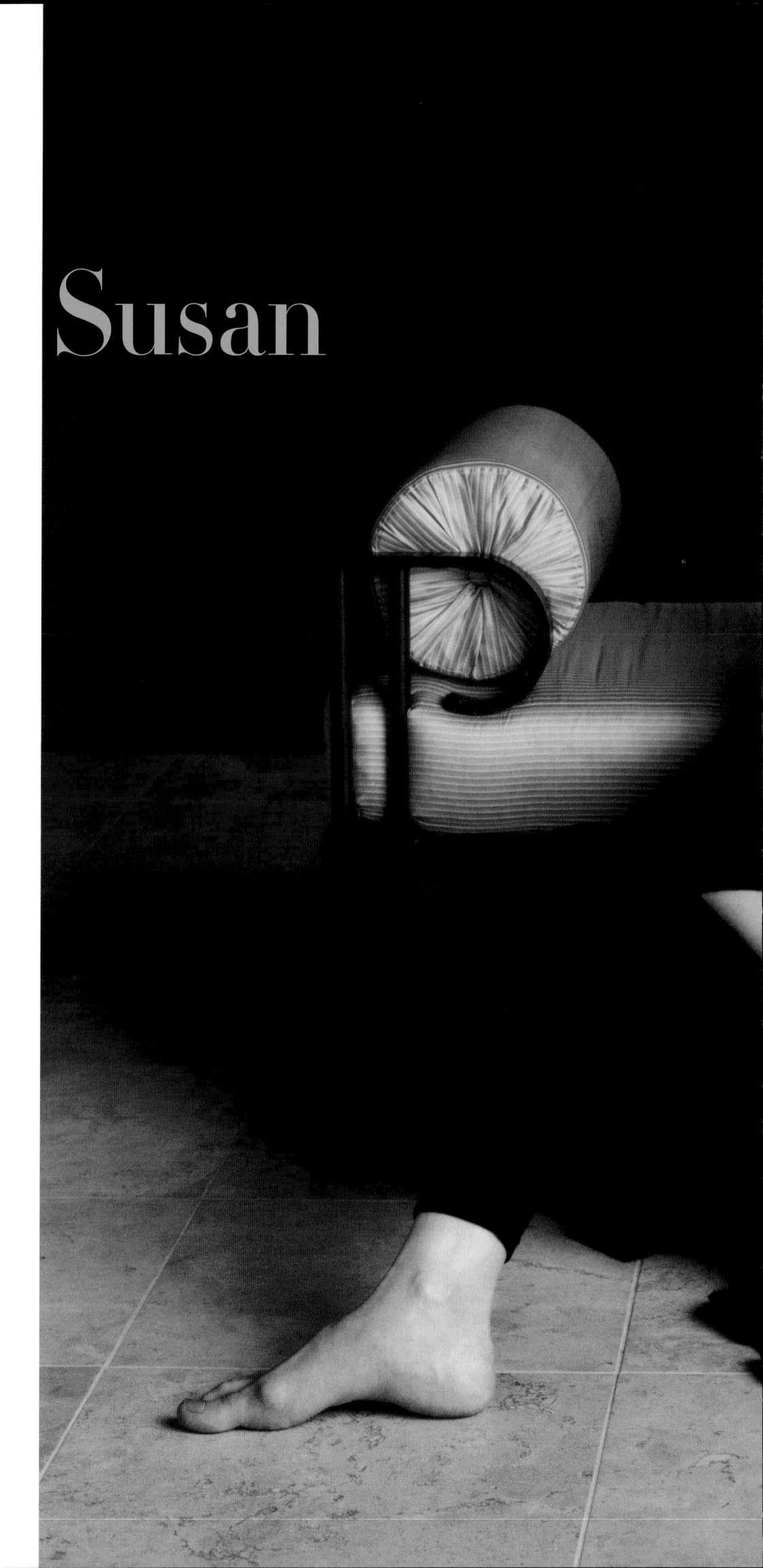

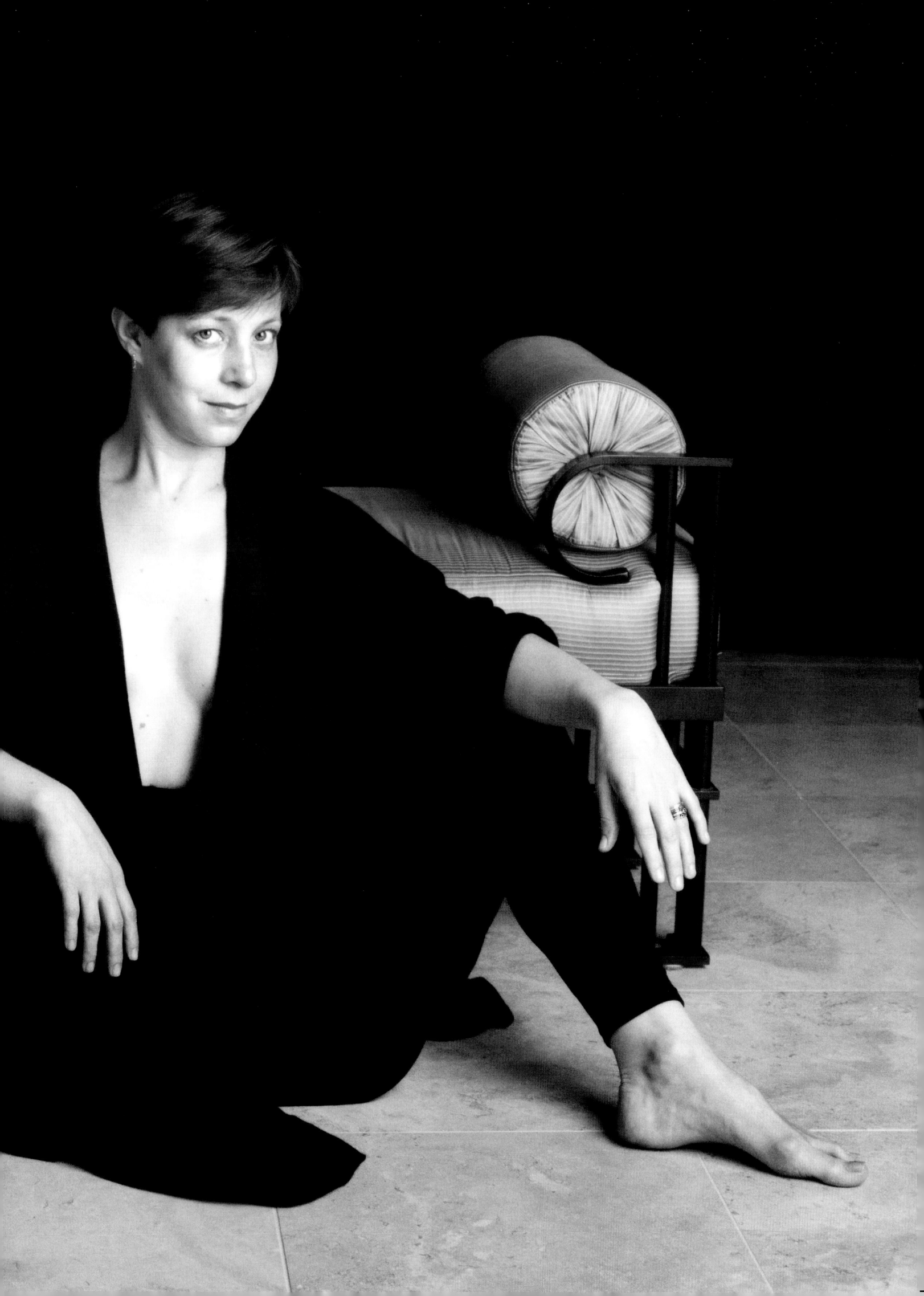

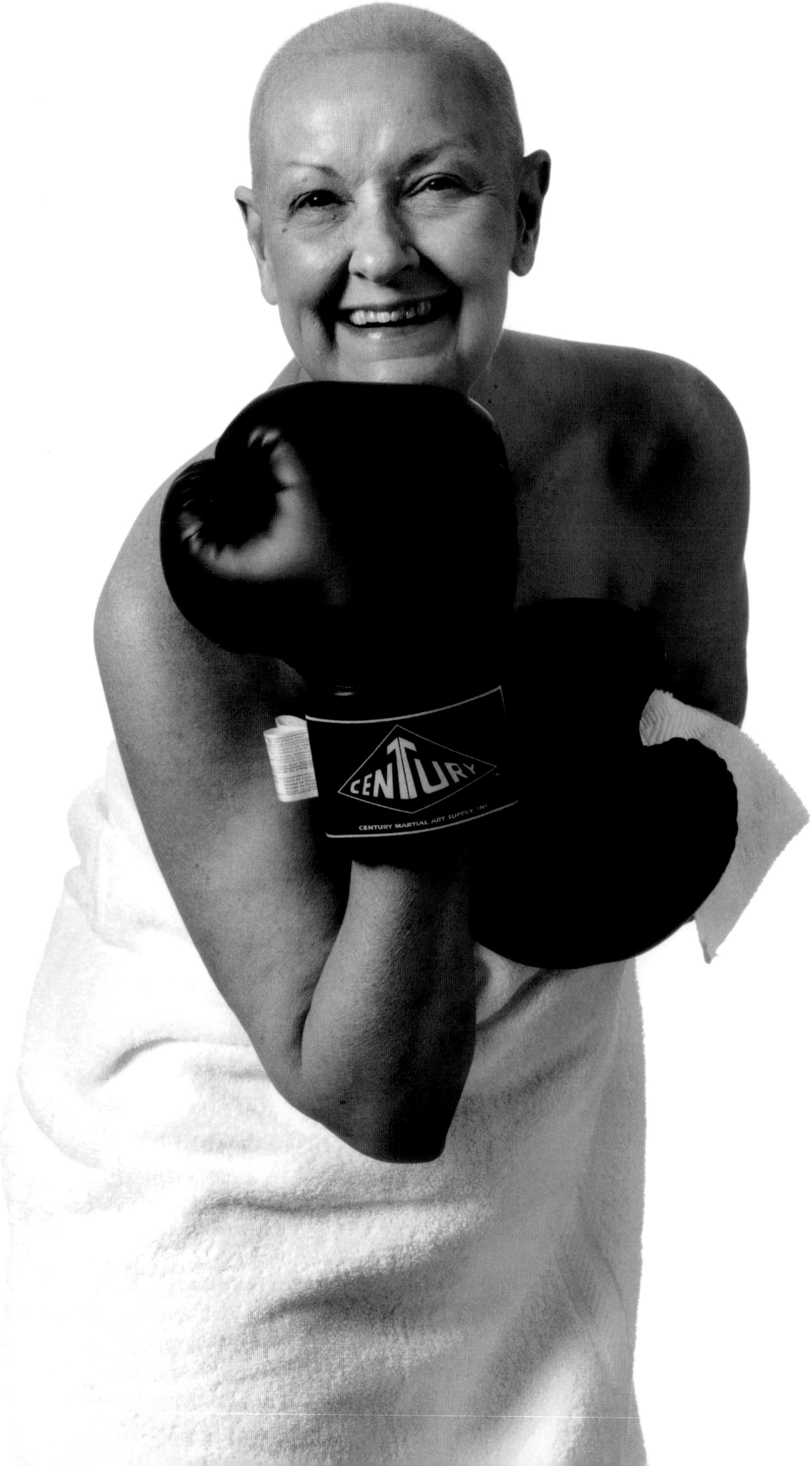
CENTURY
CENTURY MARTIAL ART SUPPLY, INC

Dana

"The first time I saw this I hated it," Dana Ravel says, pointing to her photograph. "The second time I thought, 'she got me!'" She laughs and briefly assumes the boxer's pose. But she was not always a fighter.

When her beloved husband, with whom she shared a successful art business and a passion for collecting, died after an extended illness, Dana was inconsolable. She sold their house, closed the gallery, and isolated herself from old friends. "Gene would have been so mad at me, at the way I pulled back from everything," she says.

Then she was diagnosed with breast cancer. The biopsy report, read by her sister, a Dallas pathologist, indicated that nearly all of the lymph nodes were involved. This time Dana chose to fight back. She endured the stem cell treatment recommended by her doctor. "So I made this deal with God," says Dana. "All right, God. I'll do this, but by golly, life better be interesting. I want to have fun. Life is supposed to be fun."

Two years later, she opened another art gallery. She reconnected with old friends. She did not do reconstructive surgery.

"This is your house," Dana says, thumping her chest. "Your shell, the place your soul and your mind live, you know? It's not as important as what's inside.

"Finding my peace, accepting and appreciating myself, that's the most important side effect of the cancer. Now I look in the mirror and see a friend, someone I can love. I have absolutely no fear of dying—none. But while I'm here, I want to live."

Dana died in February 2001 at the age of 57.

Monica

For Monica Yaniv, facing cancer—and life—is all about staying positive. "I don't like the word 'survivor,'" she says. "It has a negative connotation."

A scientist from Berbesheva, Israel, Monica is a Modern Hebrew instructor at the University of Texas in Austin. She was shocked at her breast cancer diagnosis in 1989 at age forty-two. Despite her family's history of breast cancer, it was not an openly discussed or widely known topic in Israel. Now at age fifty-six and having lived in the United States for more than twenty years, Monica officially fits into that category that might not have such a negative connotation after all: Survivor.

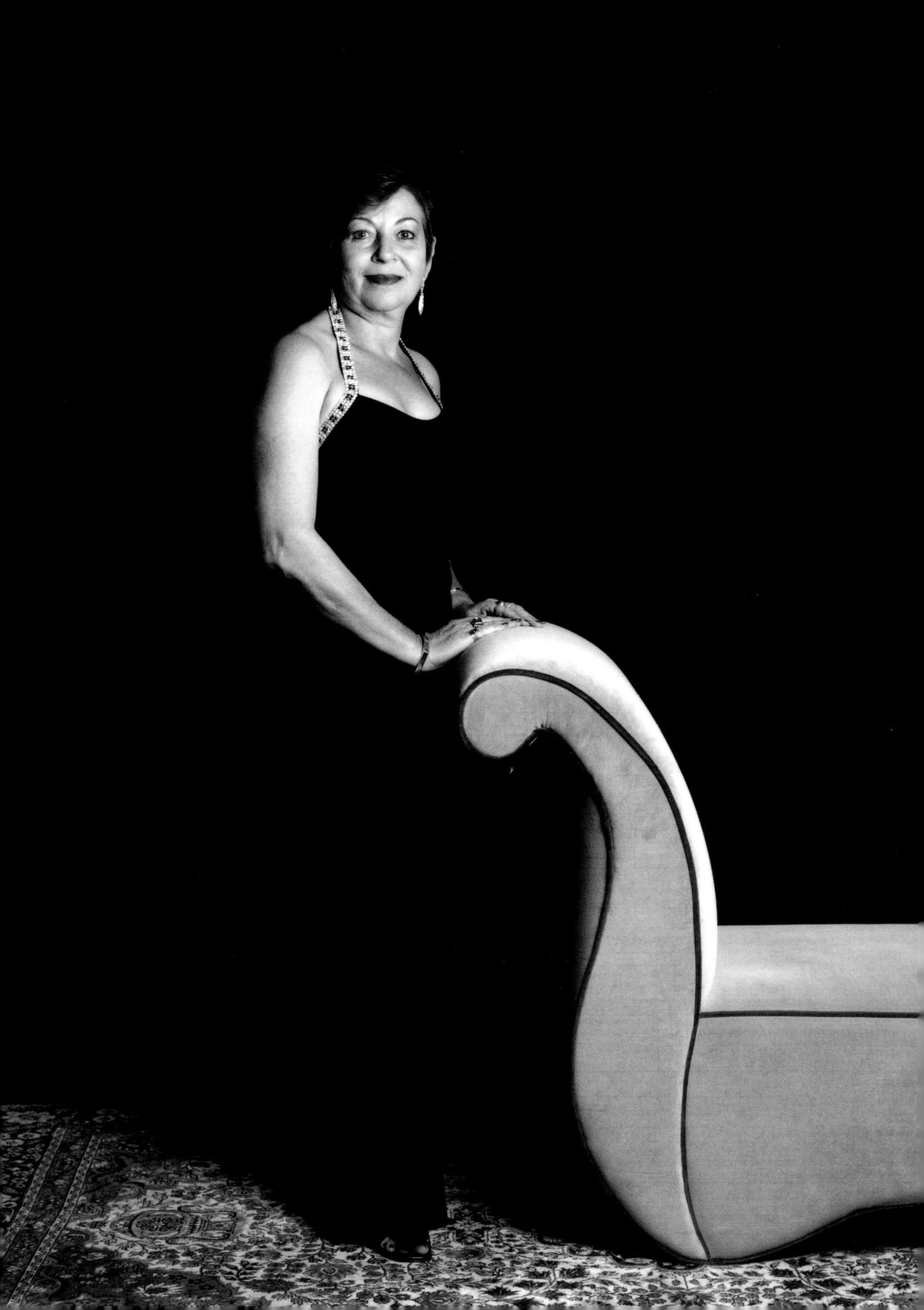

Donna and Carrie

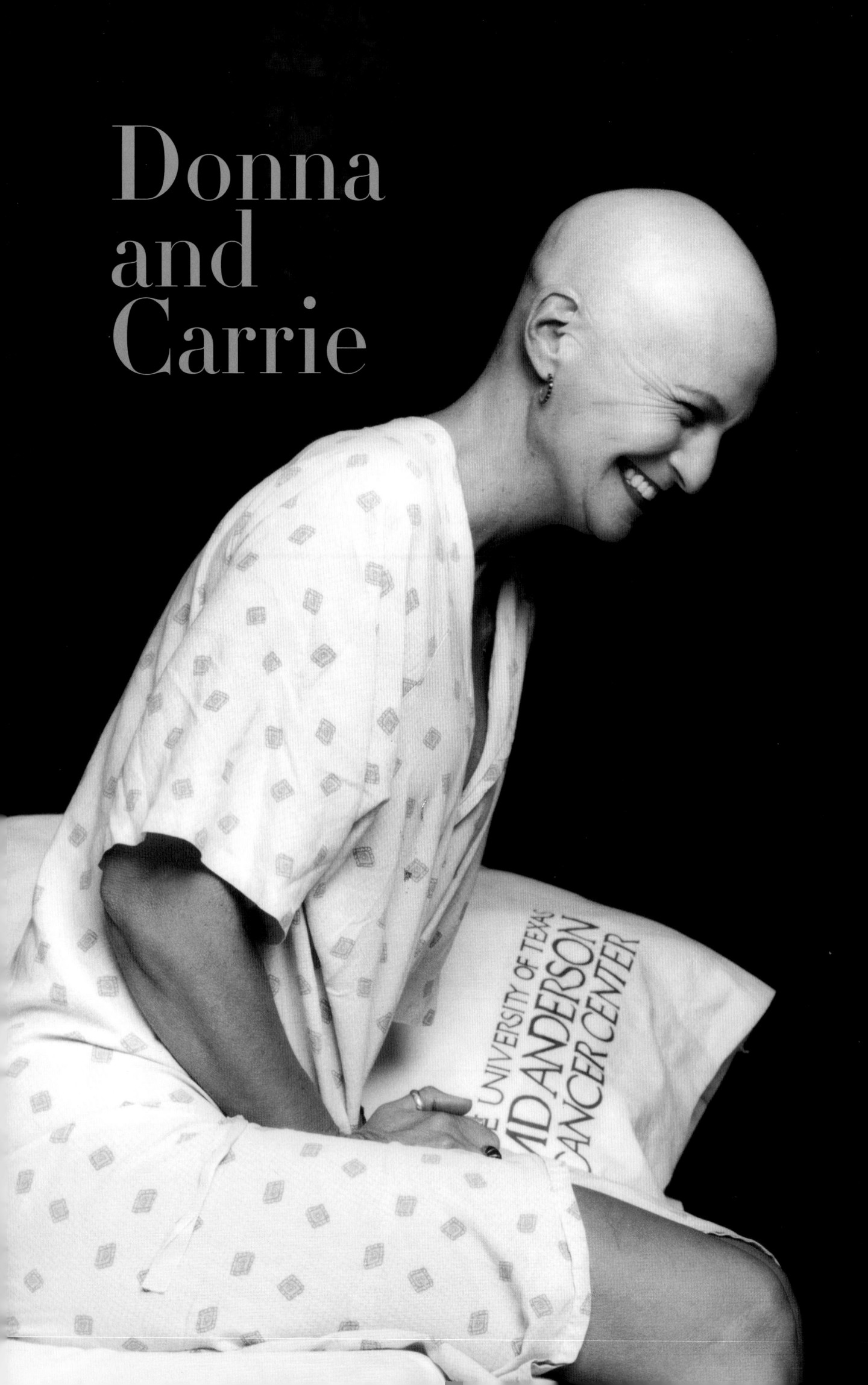

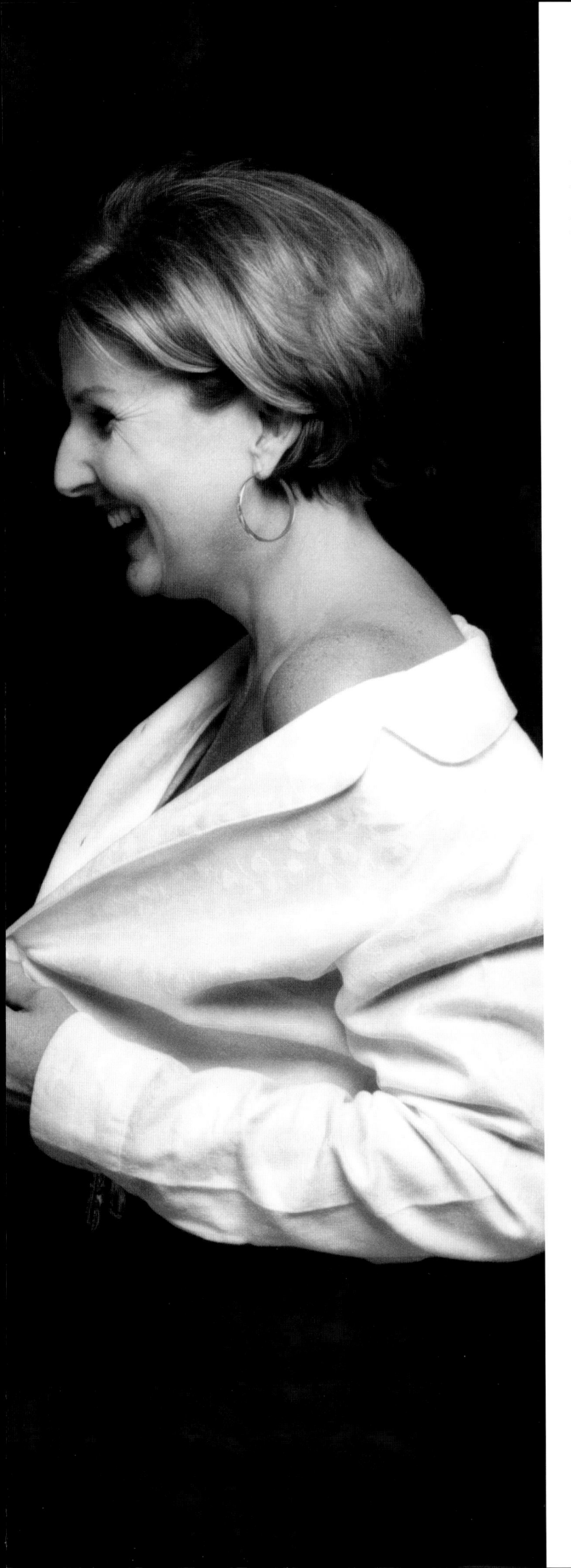

After surviving her battle with breast cancer five years ago, Carrie Wood became a volunteer at a Houston hospital, counseling breast cancer patients in the reconstruction process. There, she is part of a group called The Flashers, who show their reconstruction to and share their experiences with other women who are about to undergo the procedure. She met Donna Dohmann, with whom she is pictured playing show and tell here, through this group.

Before her diagnosis, Carrie was busy balancing her career as a senior vice president at Bank of America with her responsibilities as a wife and mother. She says she feels lucky to have gone through the experience at just thirty-nine, because it has taught her to appreciate the years ahead. She teaches her children that a good way to put their problems in perspective is to help someone else with theirs, a philosophy she demonstrates through her work at the hospital.

"Although I have walked through those doors as a very sick woman, I don't think of myself as such anymore. I now try to go through those doors to help others."

Cancer might typically be perceived as something that weakens the soul, but that was not either of these women's experience with the disease. Around the time of Donna's diagnosis, her husband left her, and she sold the hair salon she had been running for twenty-three years. "Cancer gave me the strength to survive the hurdles," she says.

Despite the major life changes Donna has been through, she says her life is falling into place and she has made a new beginning. She bought a new house in Orange, Texas, and without the confines of her salon she now has the freedom in her schedule to visit her daughter, a freshman at the University of Texas in Austin. She also has found time to volunteer for Reach for Recovery, which she describes as "the most rewarding thing I've done in my life."

Carol

Although she had little formal education, by the 1970s Carol Horn's creative side had led her to become one of five principle designers running a successful women's fashion label in New York. Since then, her travels around the world have exposed her to other cultures and influenced her designs.

When she was diagnosed with breast cancer, her focus became to take care of herself. She networked with other women fighting breast cancer, and remained fearless throughout the experience—despite the fact that her mother and aunt both shared her diagnosis. "Something's going to get me someday," she says. "But not this!"

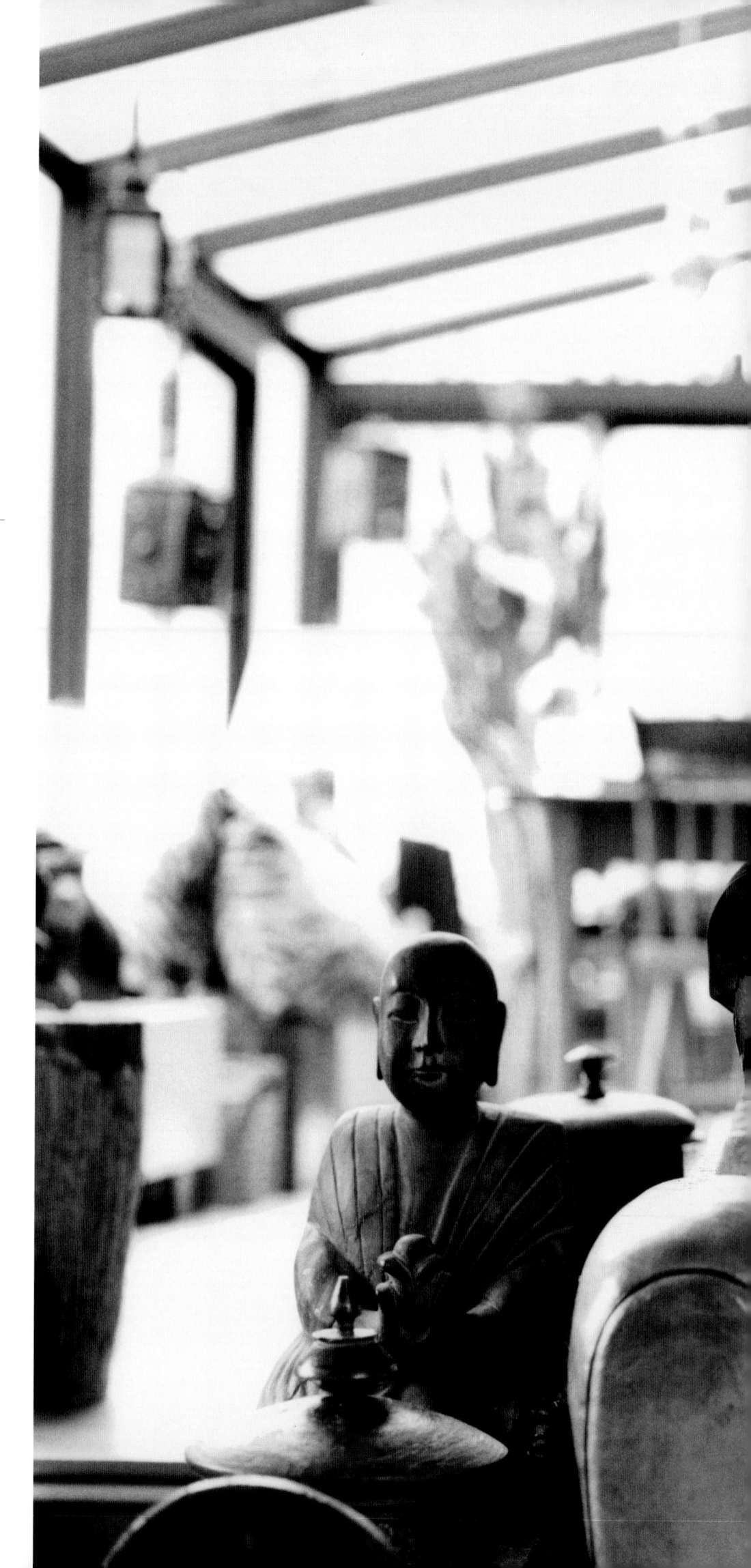

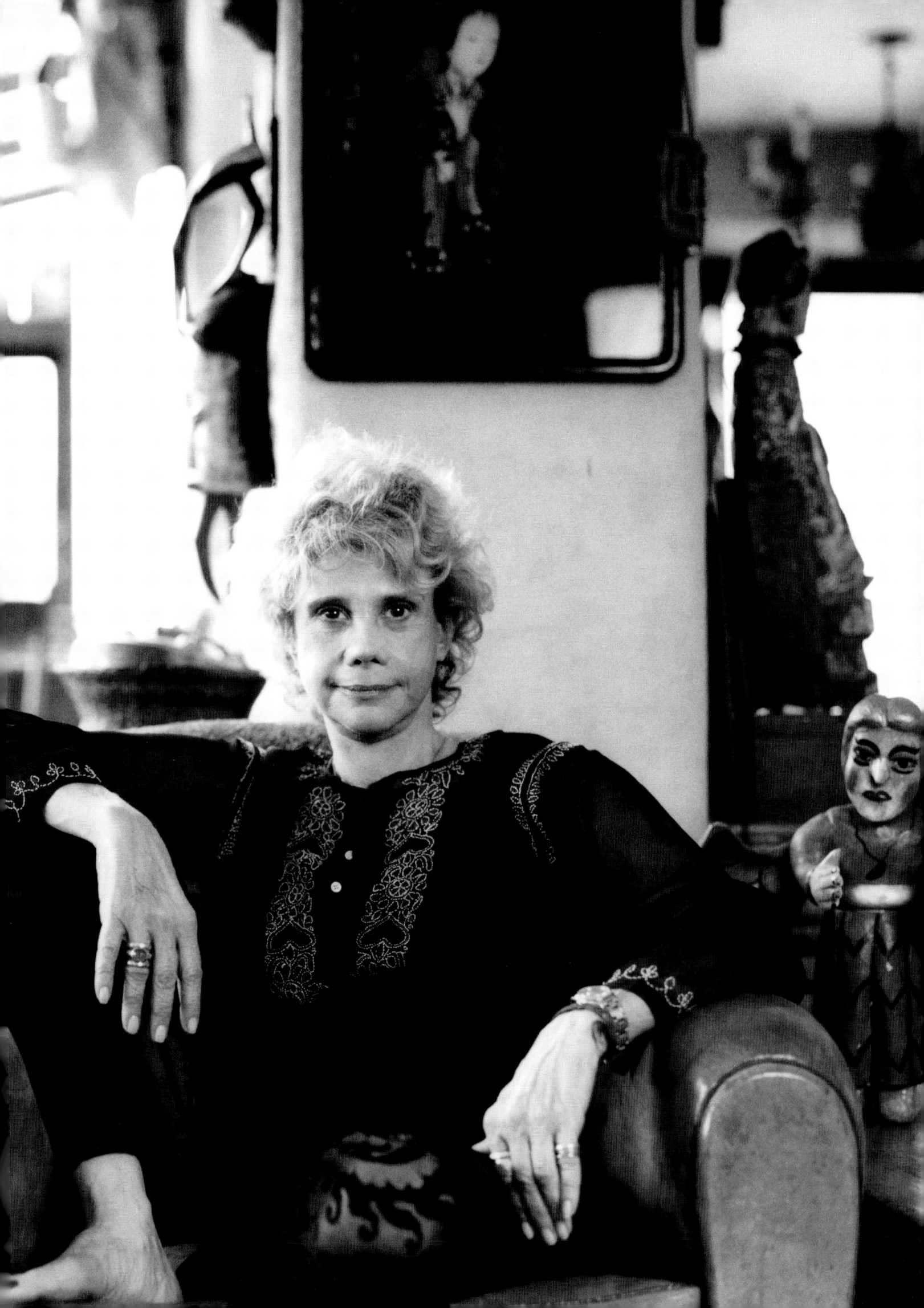

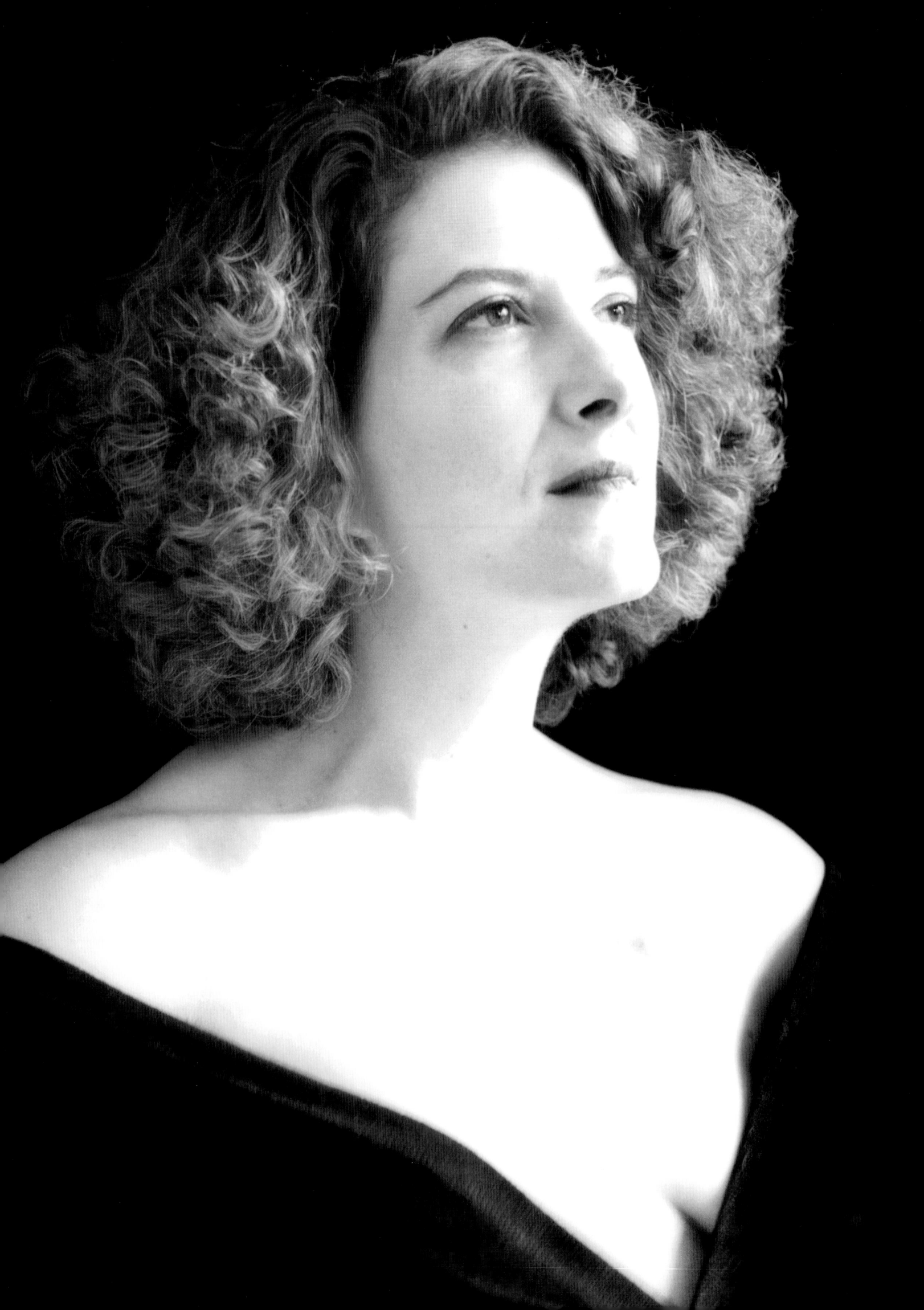

Marcy

Marcy Langer lost her ten-year battle with breast cancer in July 2001 at the age of forty, leaving behind her husband, Michael, and their son. In a letter Marcy's husband found dated September 1999, she writes:

Not even my worst enemy needs to be confronted with this horrible disease. I have found a way to create something positive out of it. I'm not a religious person, but maybe there is a master plan. My husband says, "Do you have to tell everybody you meet you have cancer?" My answer is a big "yes," because you never know who it might help.

When someone is diagnosed with cancer, it can be a very scary time. I am very outgoing and enjoy answering questions that recently diagnosed patients have. If they can be more optimistic, or more knowledgeable about their disease, then something positive has come from my breast cancer.

I live very successfully with my cancer so I don't feel sorry for myself. God must have a plan for me to try and do his work. If I can make a difference in someone's life, then it's been worth it.

Before cancer, Liz Riedel was an overworked physician's assistant who considered herself a workaholic and an insomniac. Now she sees things differently. "There's nothing worth worrying about," she says.

She and her husband live on a piece of land overlooking the Rio Grande River in New Mexico. She now spends her days harvesting and canning fruit and swimming in the river, which she views as a place for regeneration and tranquility.

Here Liz is pictured in a sandstone cave on her property. She says that with its alcoves, loft, and filtered beams of light, the cave has served as a healing sanctuary.

Liz

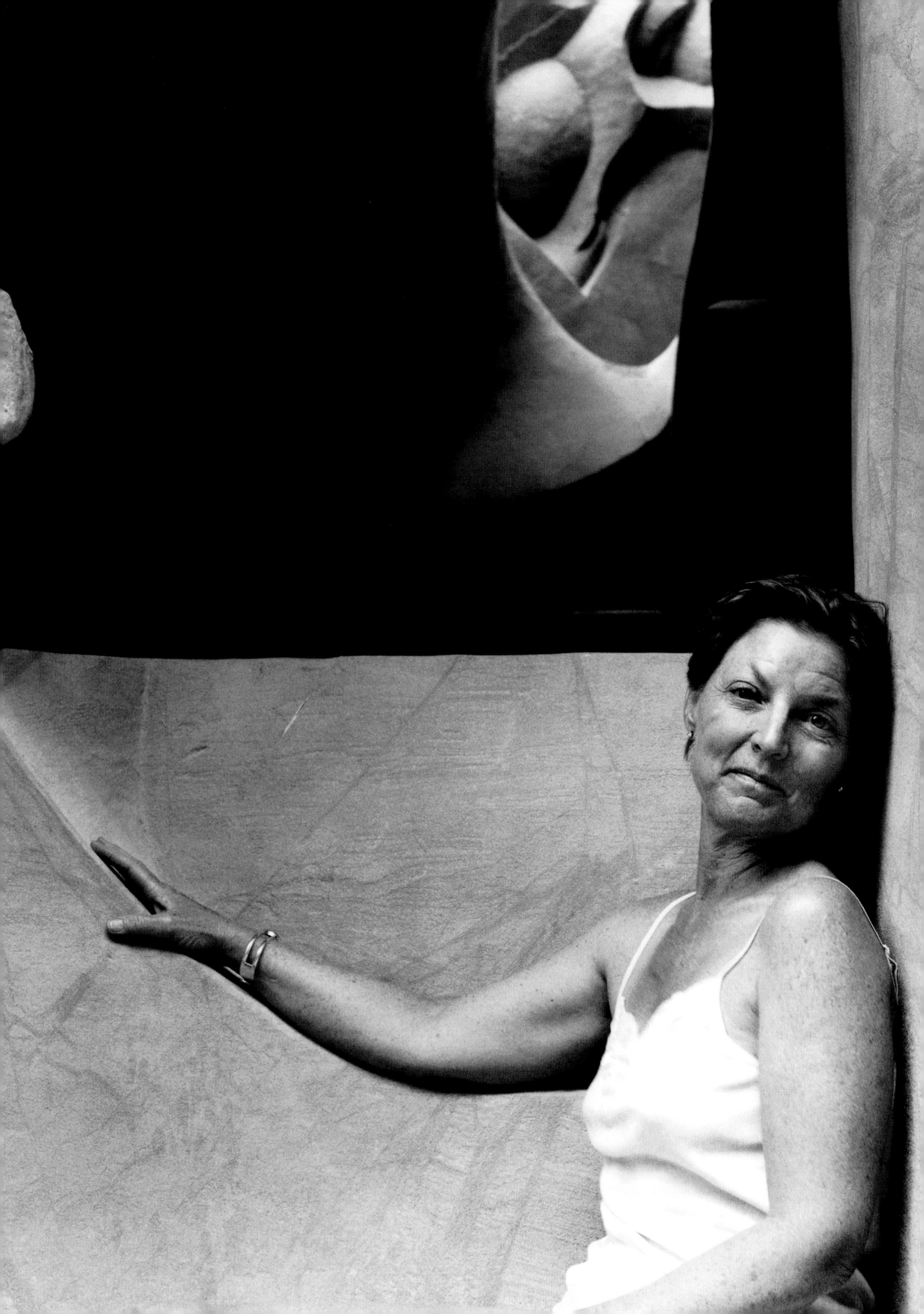

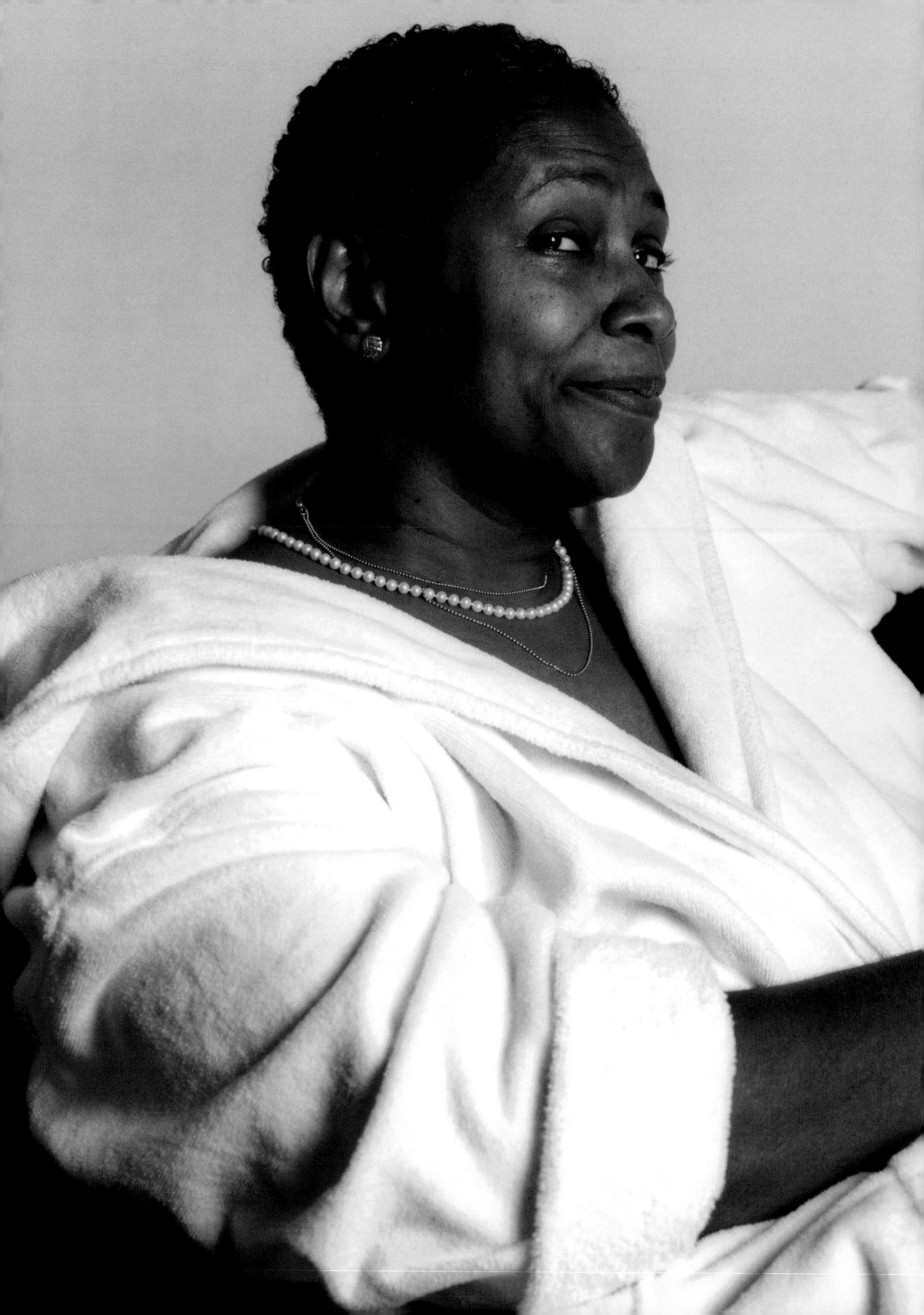

Pam

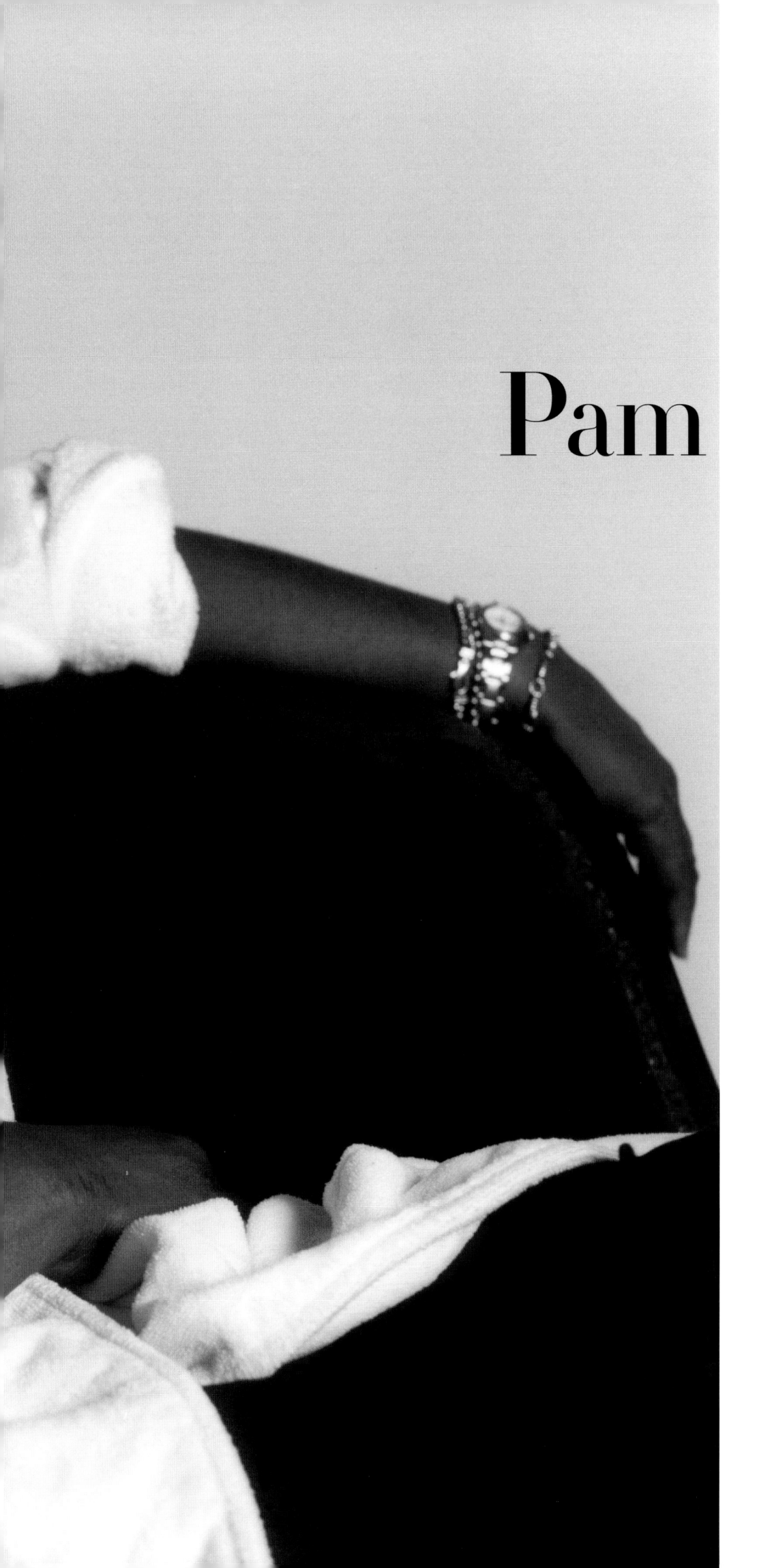

Pam Vaughn is definitely all about attitude. Before cancer, Pam was a systems programmer for twenty-five years for IBM and Arco Oil and Gas.

Cancer forced her to reevaluate her life. Before, life was about work and her hobbies, travel and racquetball. "Cancer robbed me of my joy and innocence. Being diagnosed generated feelings of guilt, shame, depression, and insecurity," she says.

As a result, she made changes and set new goals. "I went from the corporate world to an insecure mess. Support group meetings allowed me to become involved with other women."

A Kansas native now living in Dallas, Pam retired from the corporate world and dedicates her time to the Common Cares Foundation.

J.B. Pena finds solace in the garden of her Sante Fe, New Mexico, ranch, where she sits in this photo alongside what she calls her "healing wall." On the property where she lives with her husband, she rebounds from her breast cancer experience by indulging in the simple things, like riding and caring for their horses, gardening, and weaving.

Six years after her diagnosis, J.B. thinks of the disease as separate from herself. "Cancer has a mind of its own. It can raise its head at any moment in time." So it's fitting that she describes herself as adaptable. "You can take me anywhere," she says.

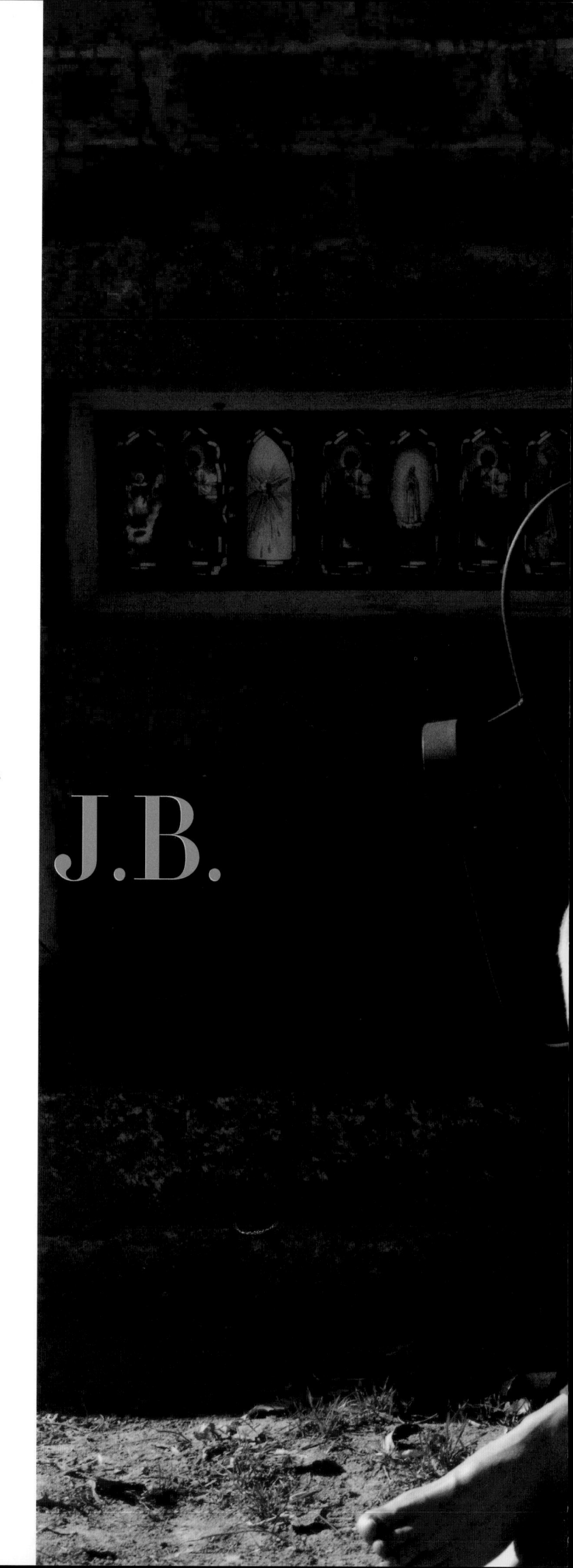

J.B.

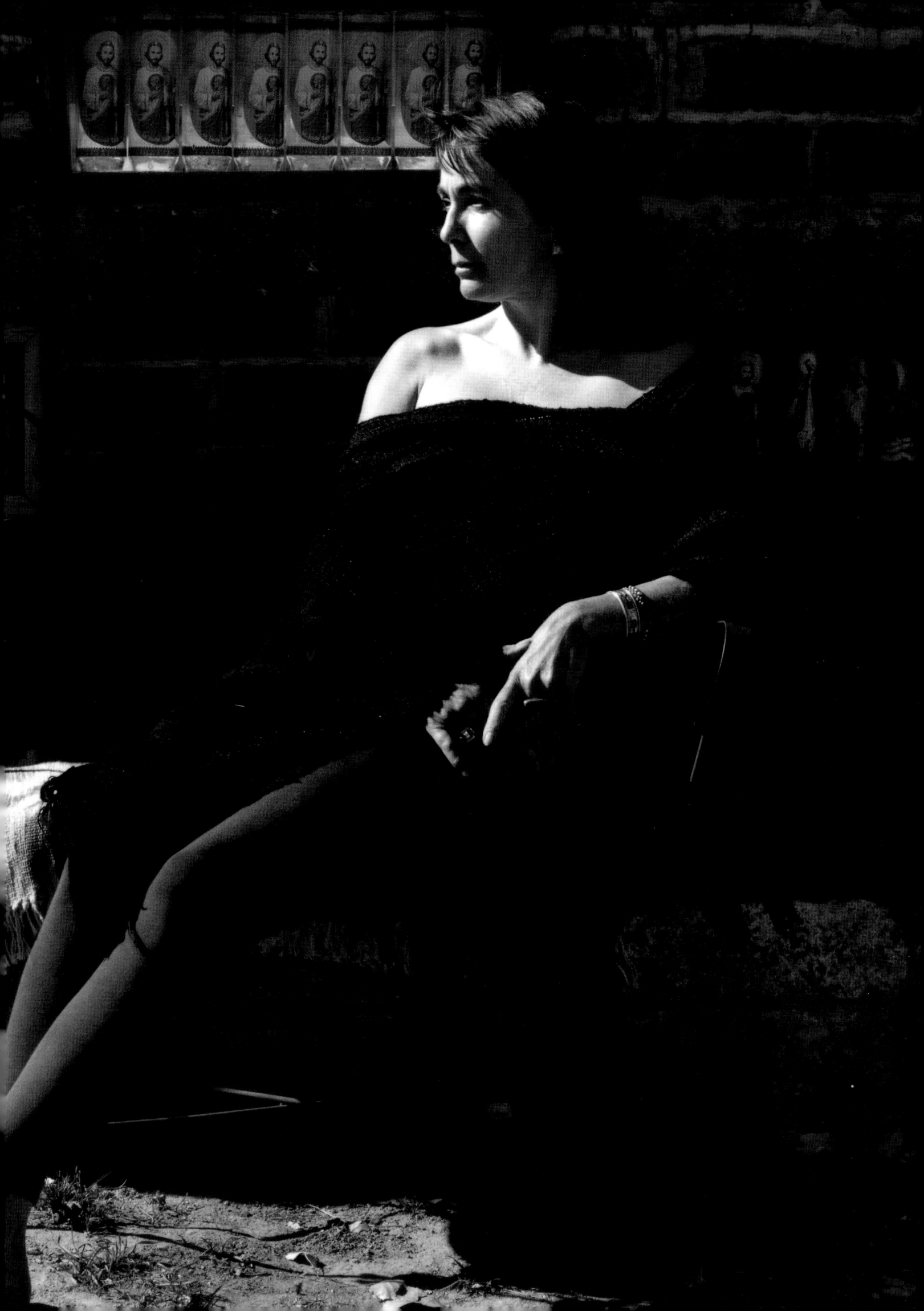

Angela and David

Angela and David Weber were diagnosed six months apart in 2001, the year they were married. Angela describes their experience together—from David going through chemotherapy on their wedding day, to the birth of their son against all odds in the spring of 2003—as mind-blowing.

"The odds of our both being diagnosed at the same time—even with male breast cancer—are unbelievable. The odds cannot be calculated. It cemented our relationship and put our lives in perspective. When something goes wrong now we say, 'Nobody died.' That's the bottom line."

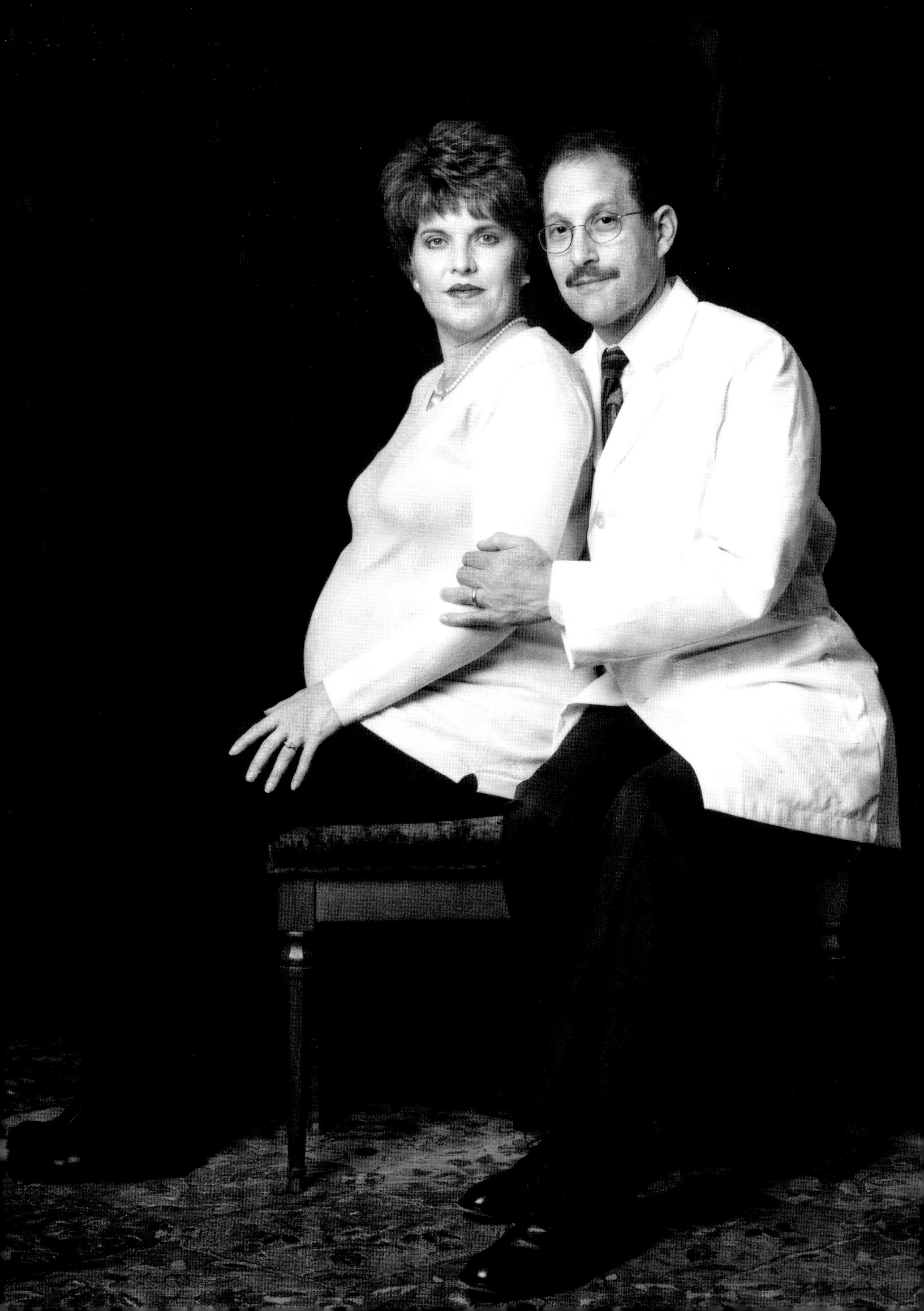

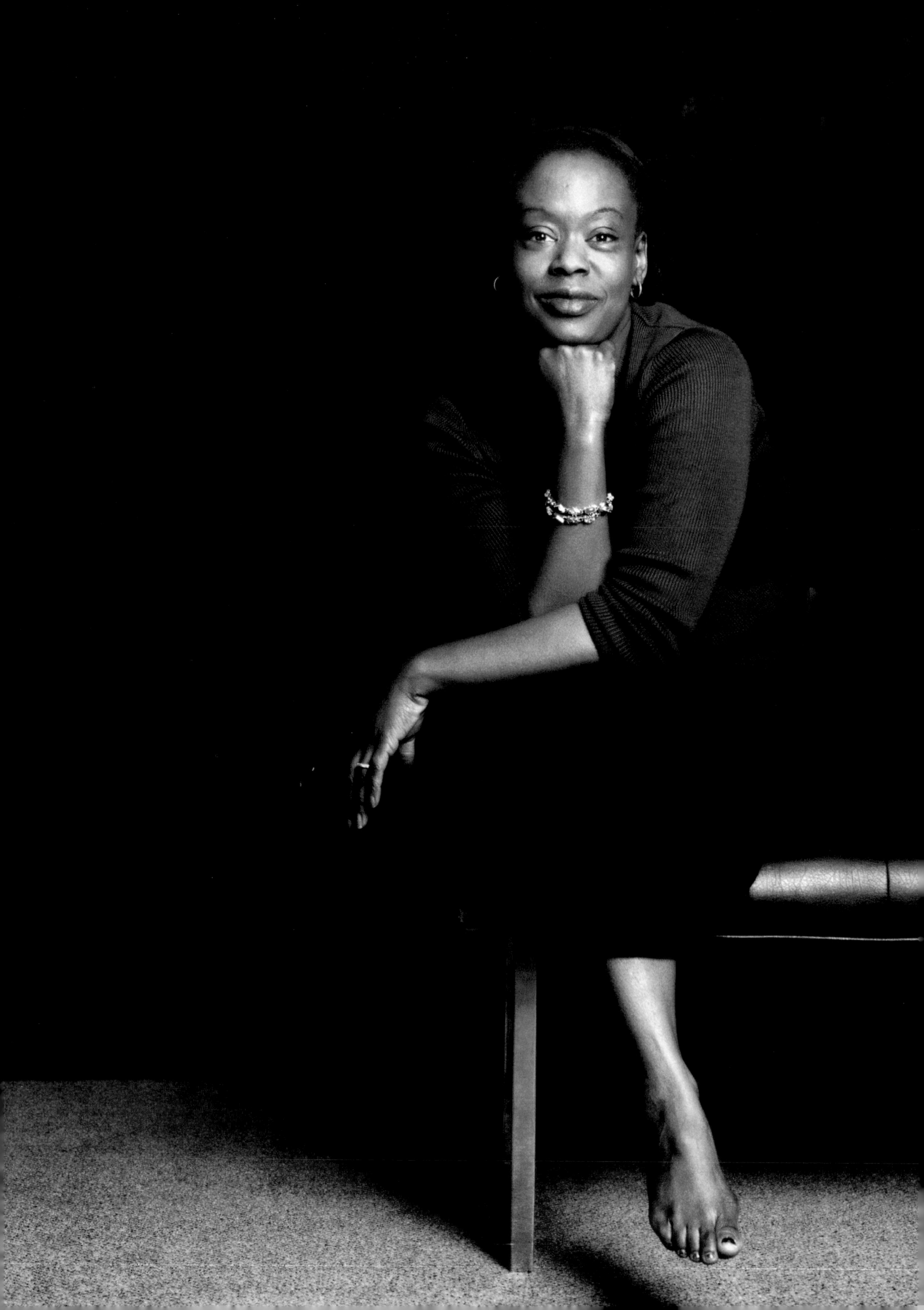

Oni

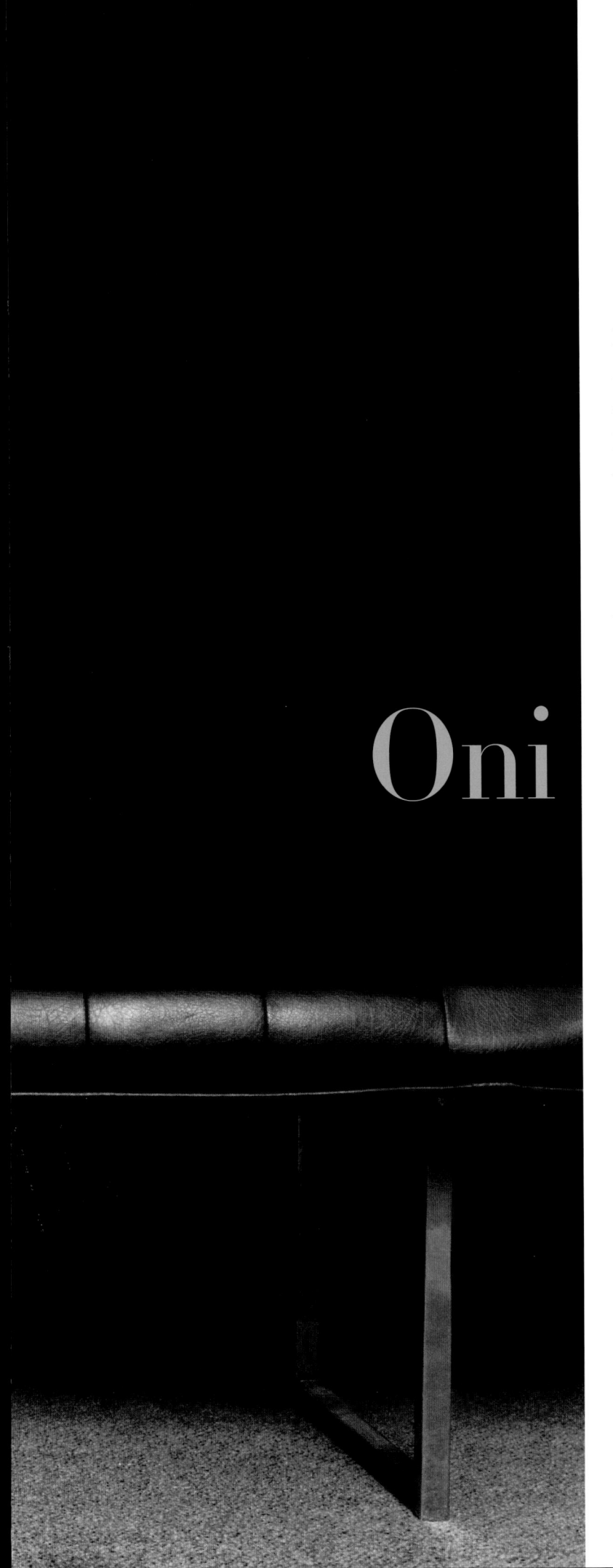

In her play titled *Tough Titty*, Oni Faida Lampley explores the emotional blow-up of a young black woman's life after a breast cancer diagnosis. The play's main character, Angela, struggles with childhood ideas about God and goodness, wrestles with the "shame of illness," and wonders what she did wrong—all while maintaining her marriage, raising two small boys, and enduring treatment. The play goes beyond having "an episode" of cancer to show what long-term survival can demand of an individual and the people who love her— and Oni's heartfelt story is powered by her firsthand experience with the disease.

Much like her character, Oni is the mother of two young boys. And also like her character, she has learned to look at cancer as a lifelong experience. "It's always going to be in my life whether or not there's a reoccurrence," she says. "I have to learn how to walk with it. It's my partner. We take turns retreating. We're in it forever."

Oni is a writer and actress living in Brooklyn, New York, who has performed both on and Off Broadway, in film, and in television commercials. Her play *The Dark Kalamazoo* recently was anthologized in *The Fire This Time: African-American Plays for the 21st Century*.

Susan Massin considers herself "the only woman to have had four breasts removed." In 1982, she elected to have a double-mastectomy and insert implants, a decision she based on her mother's early death from breast cancer at the age of forty-four. A year later, Susan's husband discovered a lump in her left breast, and this time she opted for another double-mastectomy but declined the reconstruction.

One of her most significant experiences since her recovery was participating in the Komen foundation's national run in Washington, D.C., in June 2002. "It was extremely hot, and I was soaking wet from running. Half-mile from the finish, on total impulse, no predetermined thought, I said to myself, 'This one is for me and you, Mom,' and I proceeded to flip off my tank top and run the last half-mile with my head high—focused straight ahead with a huge smile on my face and in my heart."

Susan

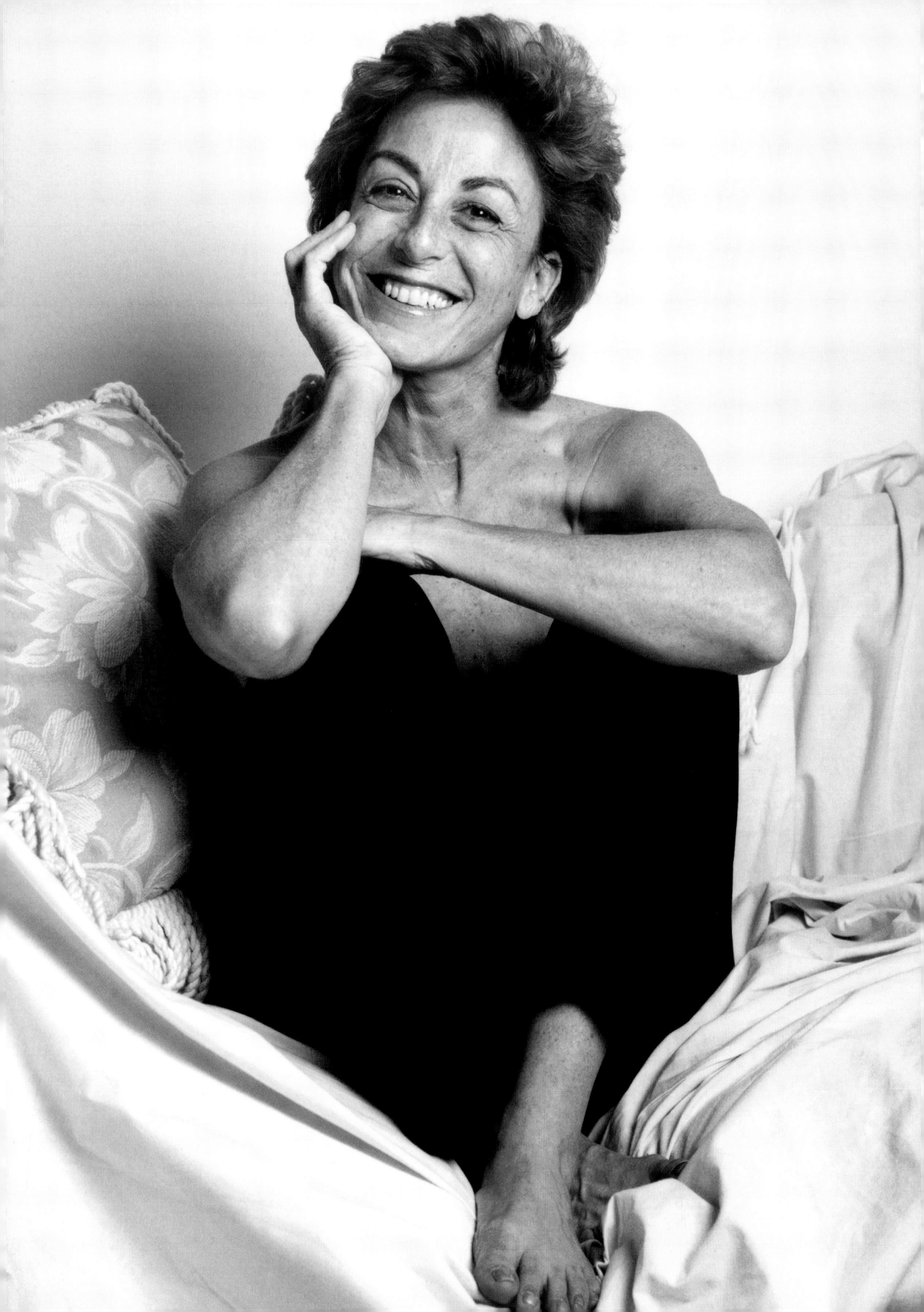

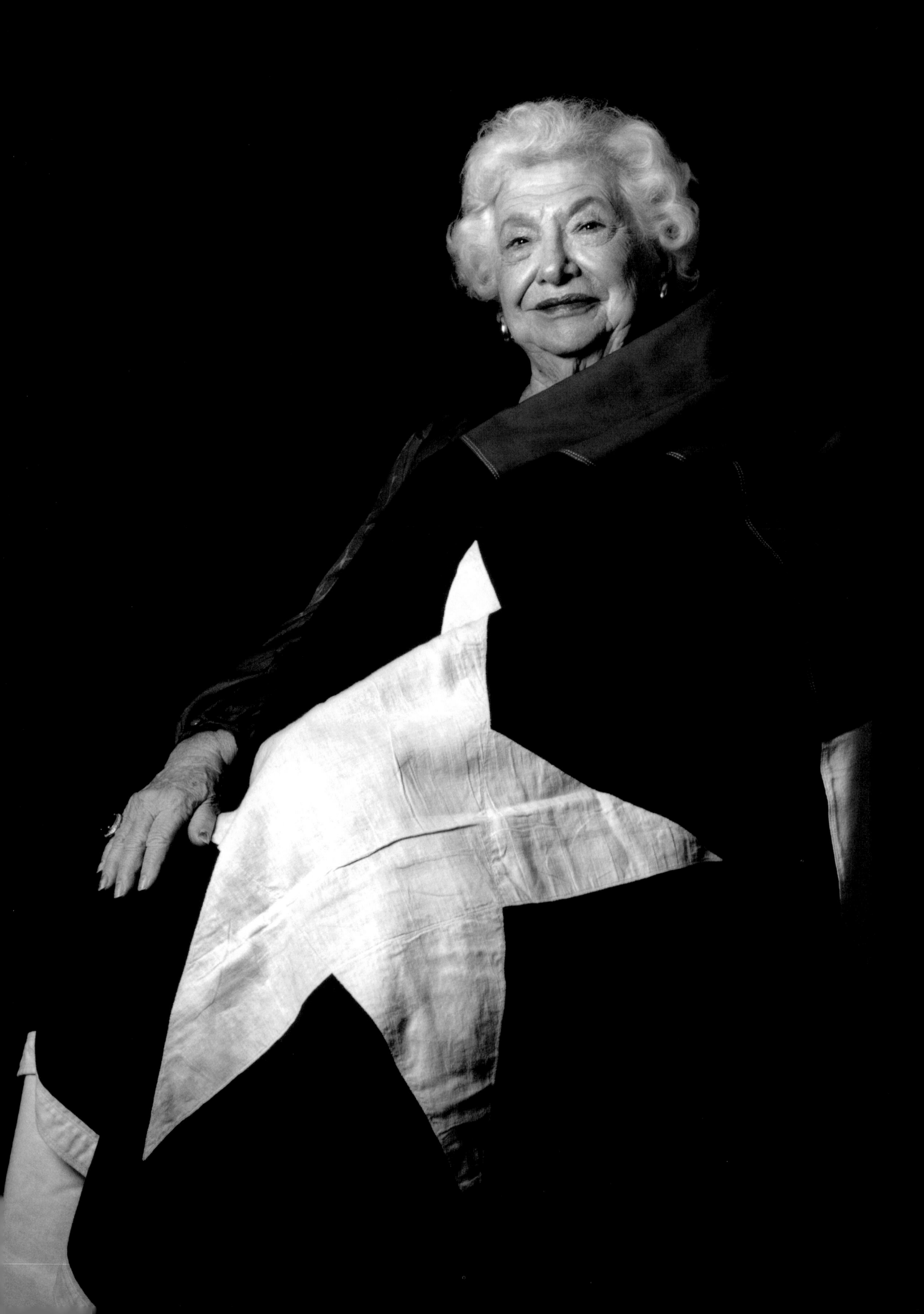

Liz

When invited to address a group on the topic of breast cancer, Liz Carpenter, author, humorist, and former press secretary to Lady Bird Johnson, delivers a prepared speech in her usual droll manner. She is otherwise hesitant to discuss her experience with cancer. "If you talk about it, it's on your mind," she says. "That 'negativeness' is bound to have its effect."

She has titled the speech "Laughing Along With Your Mastectomy," which immediately identifies its tone and desired effect. "Laughter," she insists, "is everything."

She responds quite seriously, however, when asked if there was ever a time that humor didn't work, confessing that even she has had her anxious moments. "But that shouldn't stop you from laughing. It shouldn't have to," she says. "I wanted to keep doing things." And for more than a dozen years since her surgery at age sixty-five, she has.

The Joy Luck Club

The following two images represent ten of the women who are part of the Joy Luck Club. The idea for the club was born when founding member Lucy Young (center) was recovering from breast surgery after her diagnosis in 1987. She said a prayer: "If I live to see my next birthday, I would first write a book about my experience with breast cancer, and second, start a Chinese-American organization to support and meet the needs of lonely and helpless immigrant cancer patients with language difficulties."

Both of her wishes have since been fulfilled. And today, through its affiliation with the American Cancer Society, the support group—the first Asian unit in Queens (Flushing) New York—is thriving.

FROM LEFT: WENDY LOUIE, NANCY YUEN, LUCY YOUNG, SUE LIU, ELLEN MA

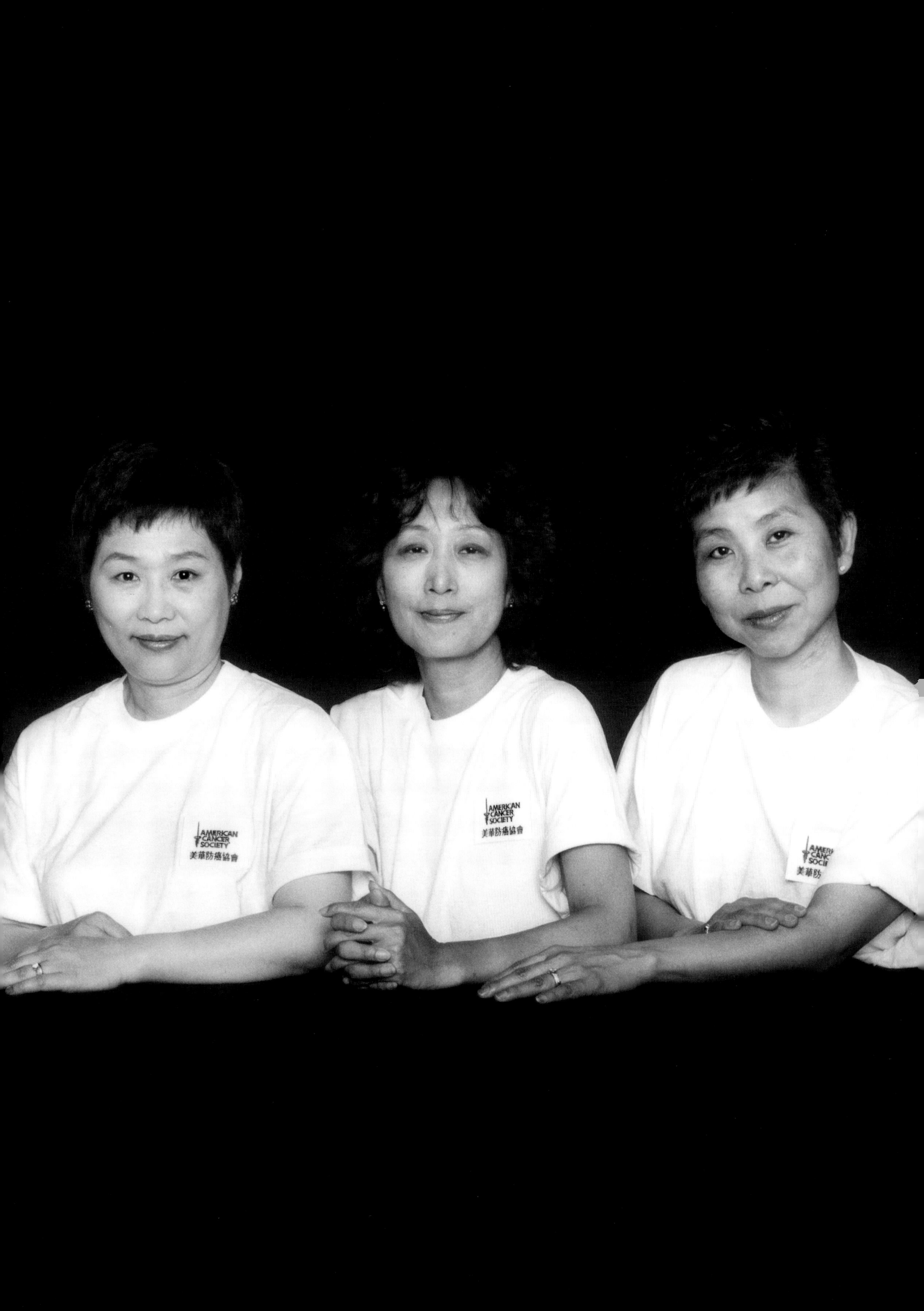
AMERICAN CANCER SOCIETY
美華防癌協會
AMERICAN CANCER SOCIETY
美華防癌協會

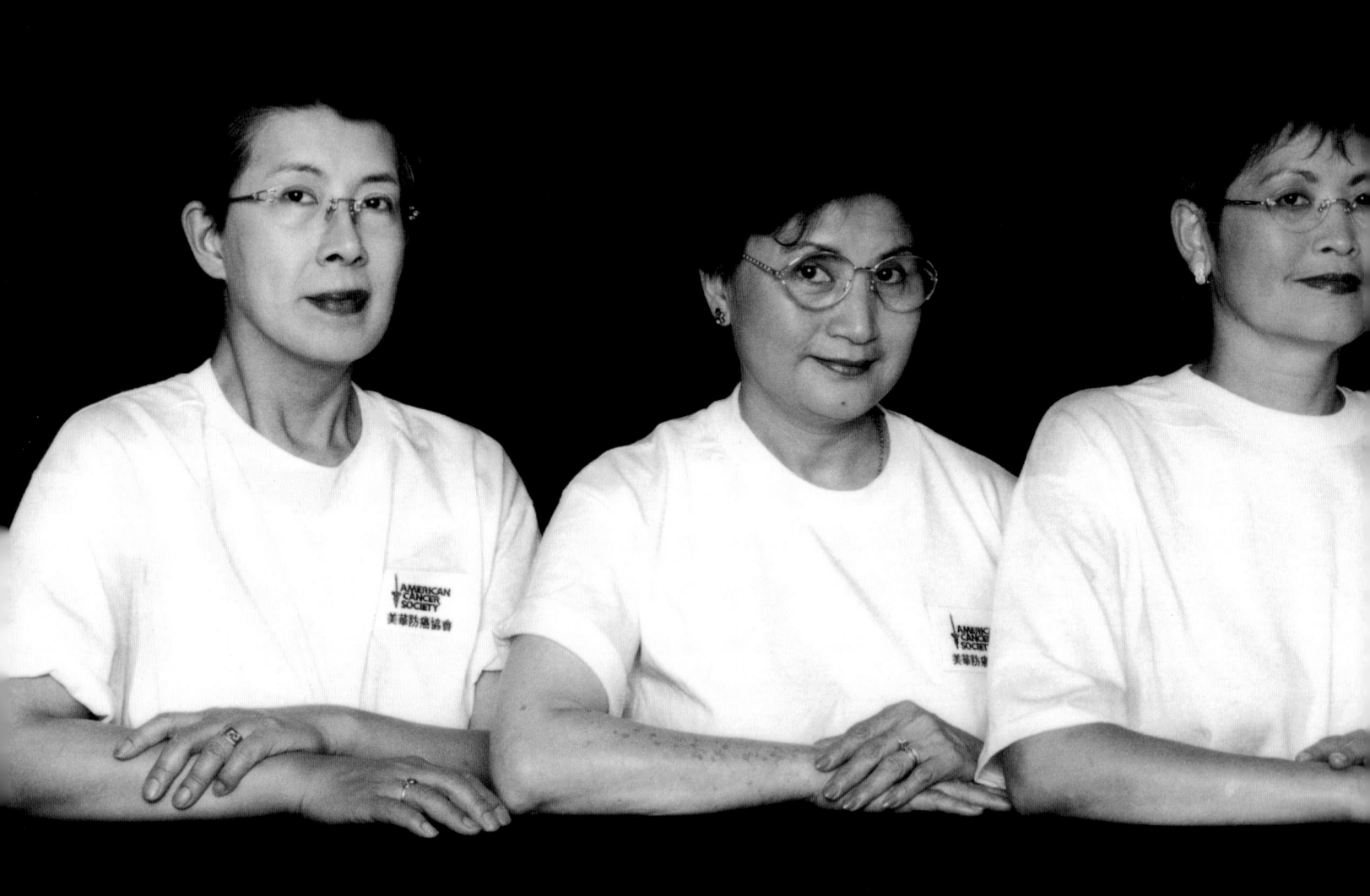

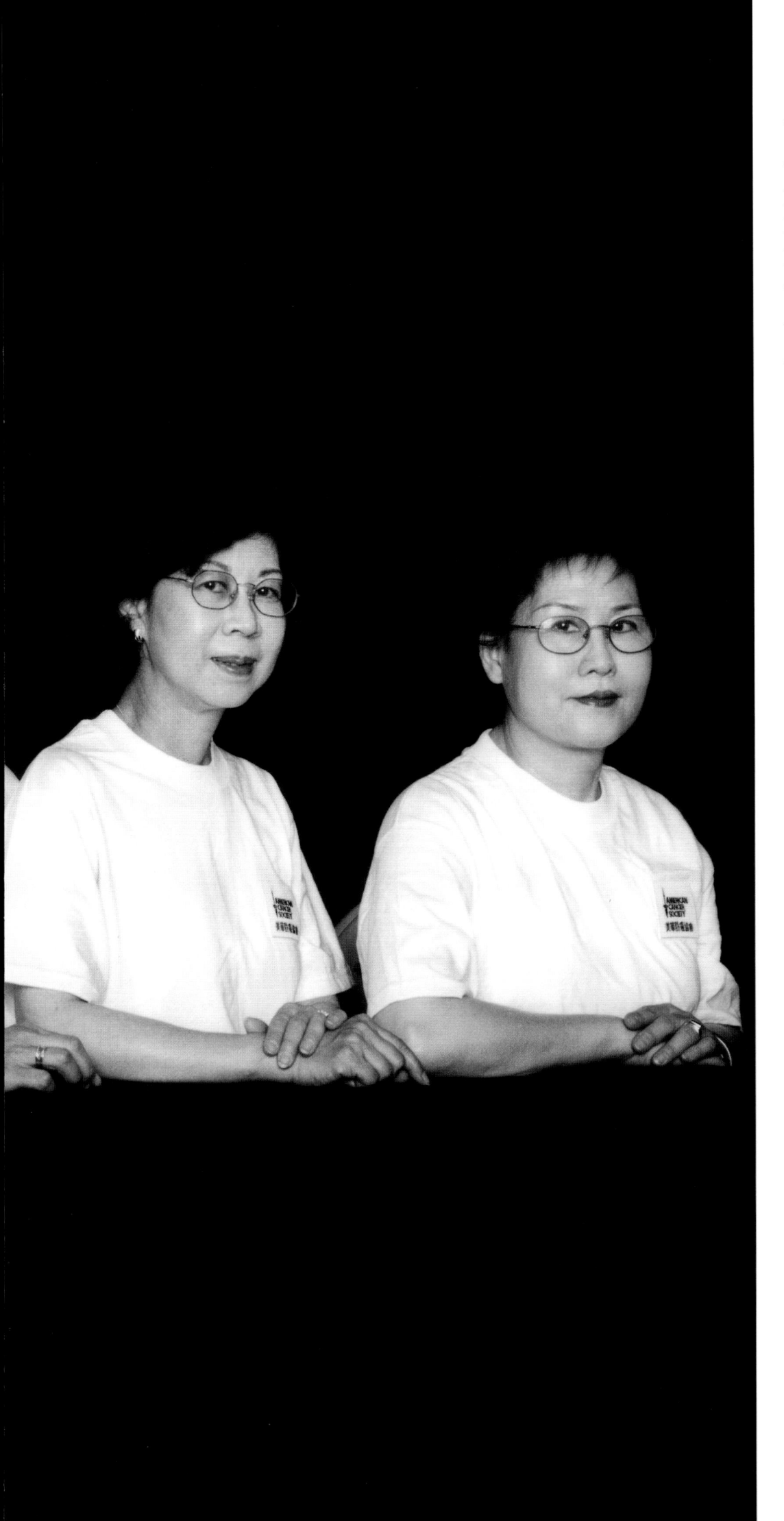

The women of the Joy Luck Club are proactive—doctors, lawyers, business leaders, housewives. They get together weekly for support and a connection—they share their joy for life.

From left: May Eng, Sanly Lamb, Dr. Jyming Wang, Joanna Leung, Betty Lee

Marty

Marty Leonard says she has always felt blessed, despite her two breast cancer diagnoses in the past thirteen years. She devotes her time to a number of worthy causes, including the United Way, the Junior League, and her local hospital's cancer center. For the past forty-two years, she has worked in developing and supporting the Lena Pope Orphanage and Children's Home in Fort Worth, Texas. Here she is pictured in the home's Marty Leonard Community Chapel, which was a surprise fiftieth birthday gift from her family and friends to honor her longtime commitment to the home. Marty also carries on the legacy of her father, a developer of country clubs nationwide, in orchestrating the building of a Nike Research Center for golf.

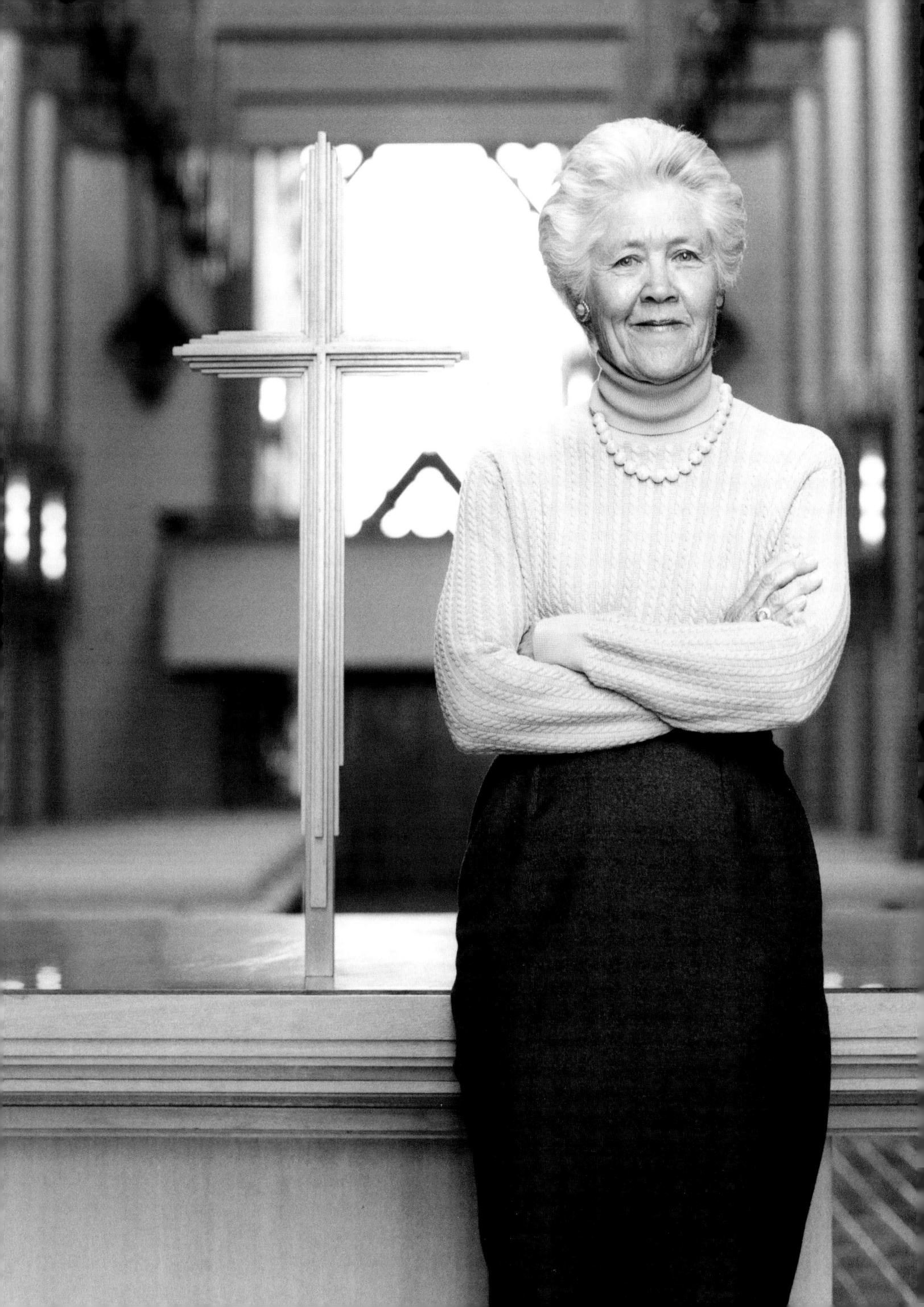

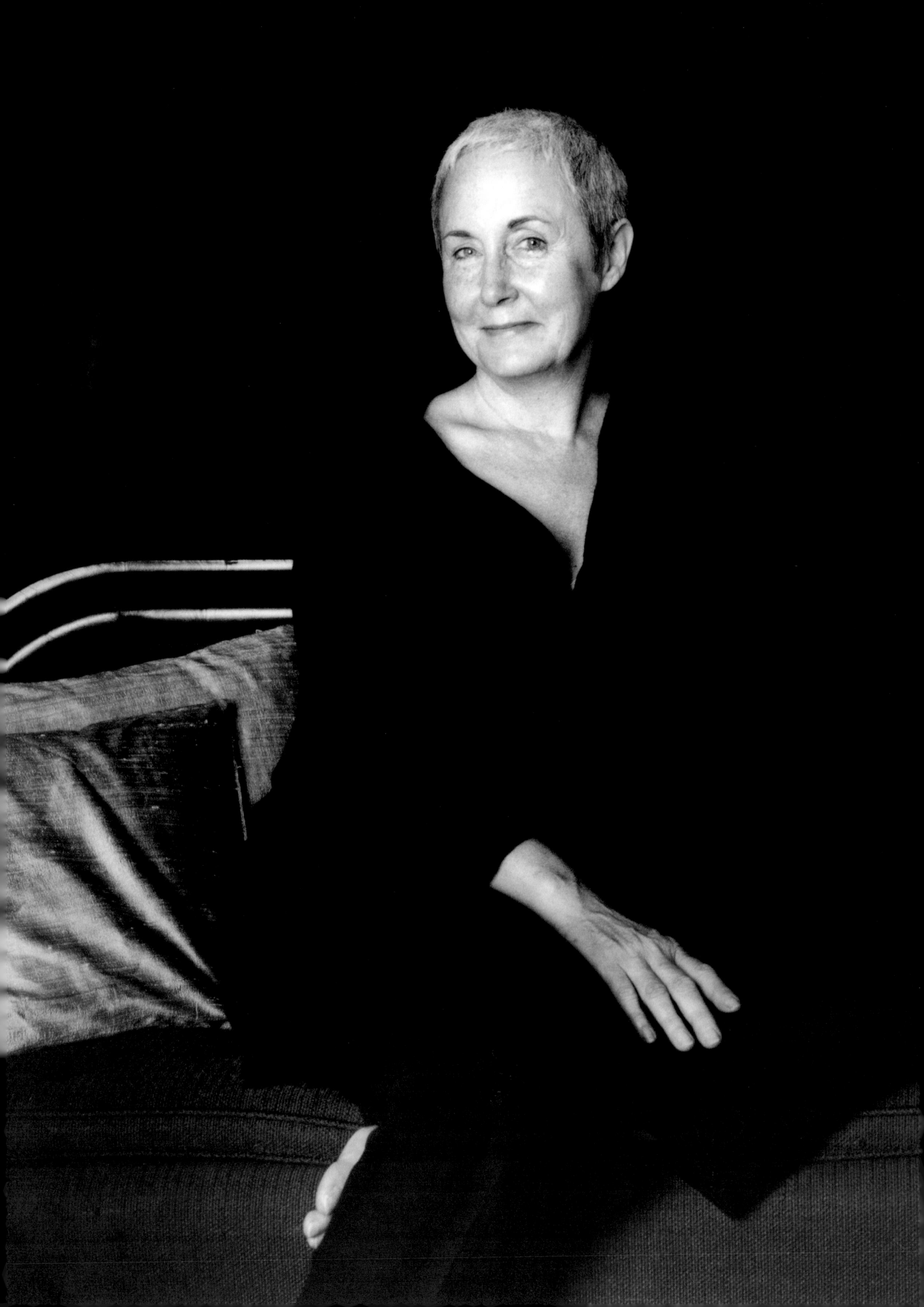

Phoebe

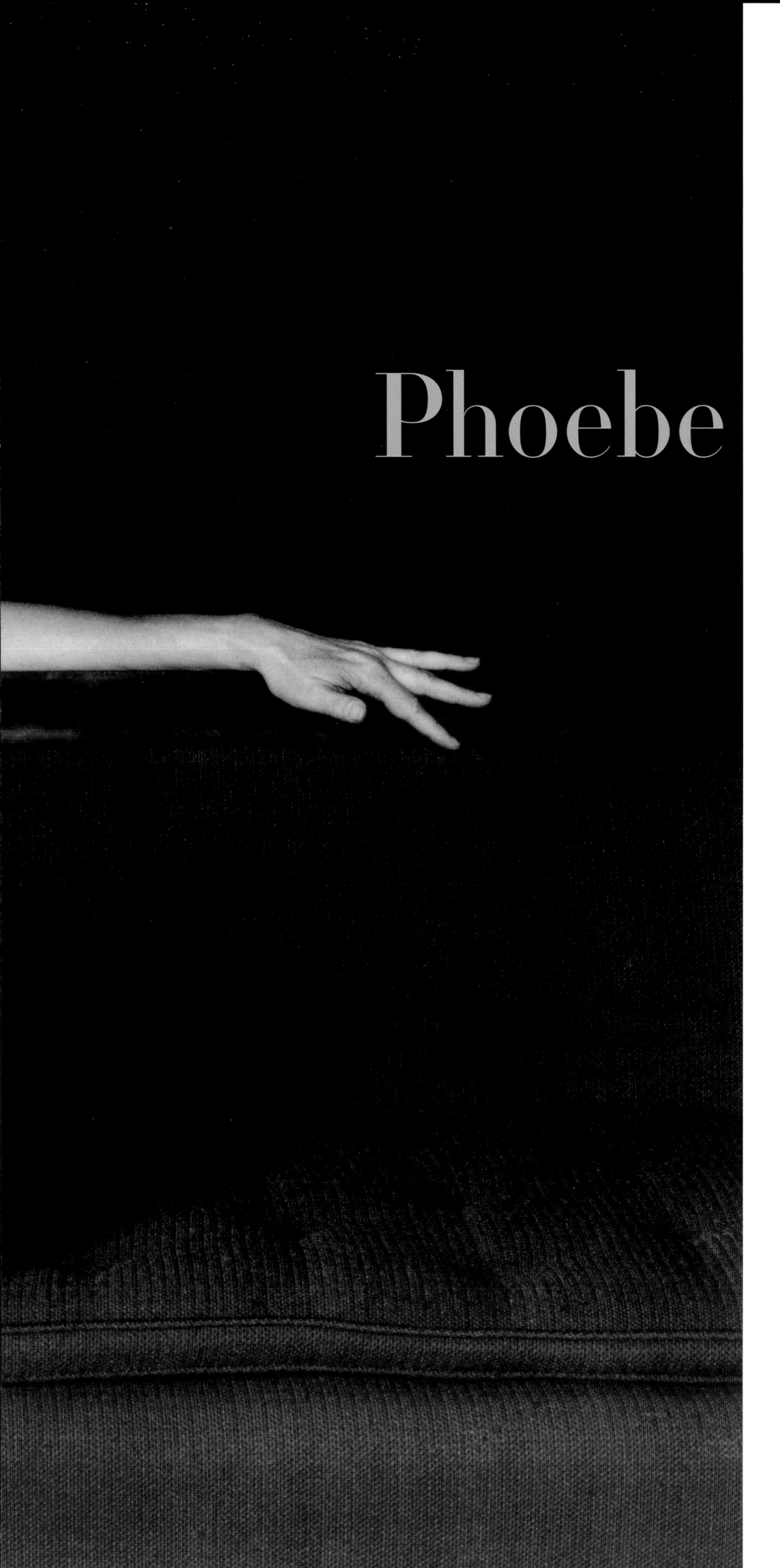

Losing her hair during chemotherapy cured Phoebe Wood of the ritual of dying her hair—and she found that she loves her hair short. Phoebe has owned a framing shop in Jenkintown, a suburb of Philadelphia, for twenty-seven years. She always used to put her disease in perspective by saying, "My cancer is about as easy as a broken arm." Coincidentally, three years later she did break her arm—and with the many orthopedic surgeries that followed, she found that cancer had actually been the easier of the two ordeals.

Mary

"In a way, my breast cancer has been tied to my work as a journalist," says Mary Walsh, who has won two Emmy Awards and two Dupont Awards from Columbia University since her diagnosis. "I cover national security, and the doctors first told me there was a serious possibility that I had cancer on September 10, 2001. So when terrorists attacked the United States on 9/11, I was launching on the most important story of my professional life just as I launched the most important battle of my personal life. I won both—my first Dupont was awarded the day after I completed my radiation.

"Two years later my cancer reoccurred, and I had to go through the physically and emotionally painful ordeal of having a mastectomy. Once again, I won a Dupont—this one for coverage of the war in Iraq. Usually I keep my head down—just do my work and take quiet satisfaction in what I've accomplished. Thinking about facing down breast cancer along with the awards I've won for my work, however, is the only time I truly allow myself to be proud. It's a 'say it loud' moment. I'm proud, damn proud of being a cancer survivor. And damn proud of the Emmys and Duponts."

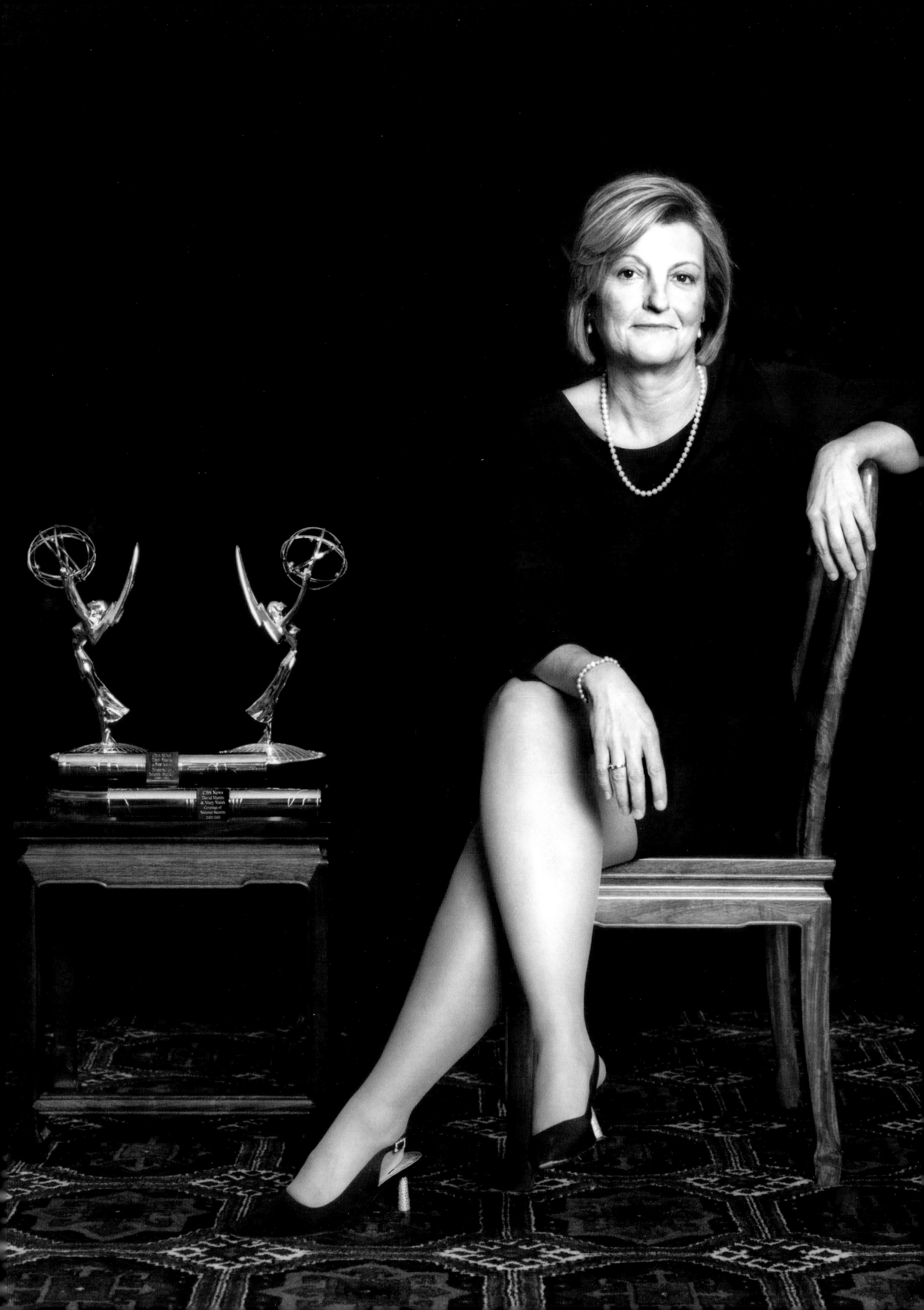
CBS News
David Martin
& Mary Walsh
Coverage of
National Security

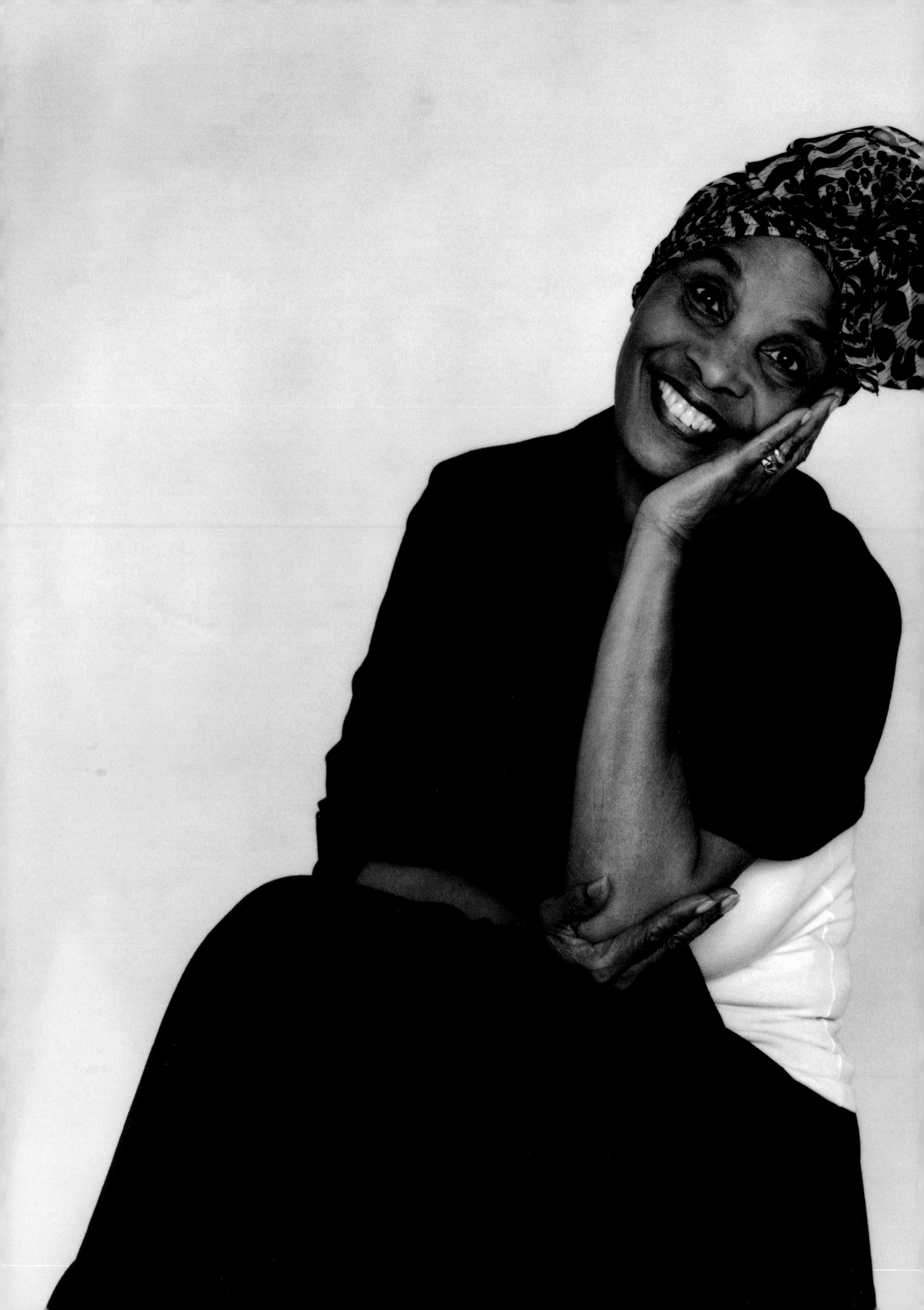

Pearle

When Pearle Griffith-Eccles was diagnosed with breast cancer in 1972, her thoughts were consumed with her two-year-old son. "I prayed to see my son finish high school," she says. "I never asked about college—just high school. I still remember [graduation] day. I was so happy." Today, she is still enjoying more than thirty years of motherhood, coupled with forty years of marriage to her husband, Errol.

A registered nurse in New York City, Pearl helps educate and care for other women with breast cancer and other health problems daily—but she doesn't stop there. She literally volunteers every single day, whether it's in a support group helping mothers heal from bereavement, visiting a hospice, working with a local school for the deaf, or even traveling to the Caribbean to teach women there about preventing and detecting breast cancer.

Gayle

A self-described "uncomplicated" mother, wife, and equestrian, Gayle Clark was initially diagnosed with breast cancer in 1998, then again in 2001. When she was injured during a horseback-riding accident in 2003, cancer was detected in her liver and other areas.

Gayle says she has never considered herself "sick" or felt that her life diminished in any way while dealing with cancer. She deals with the disease by doing her best not to let it interfere with her life—she finds riding therapeutic and relies on her family and her faith to help her stay strong. "My husband and I love to ride together," she says. "Hopefully into the sunset together."

Here she is pictured with friends from the equestrian center who shaved their heads to support her through chemotherapy.

From left: Linda Hoffman, Gayle (on the horse), Patrick Lyons, and Renee Albrecq

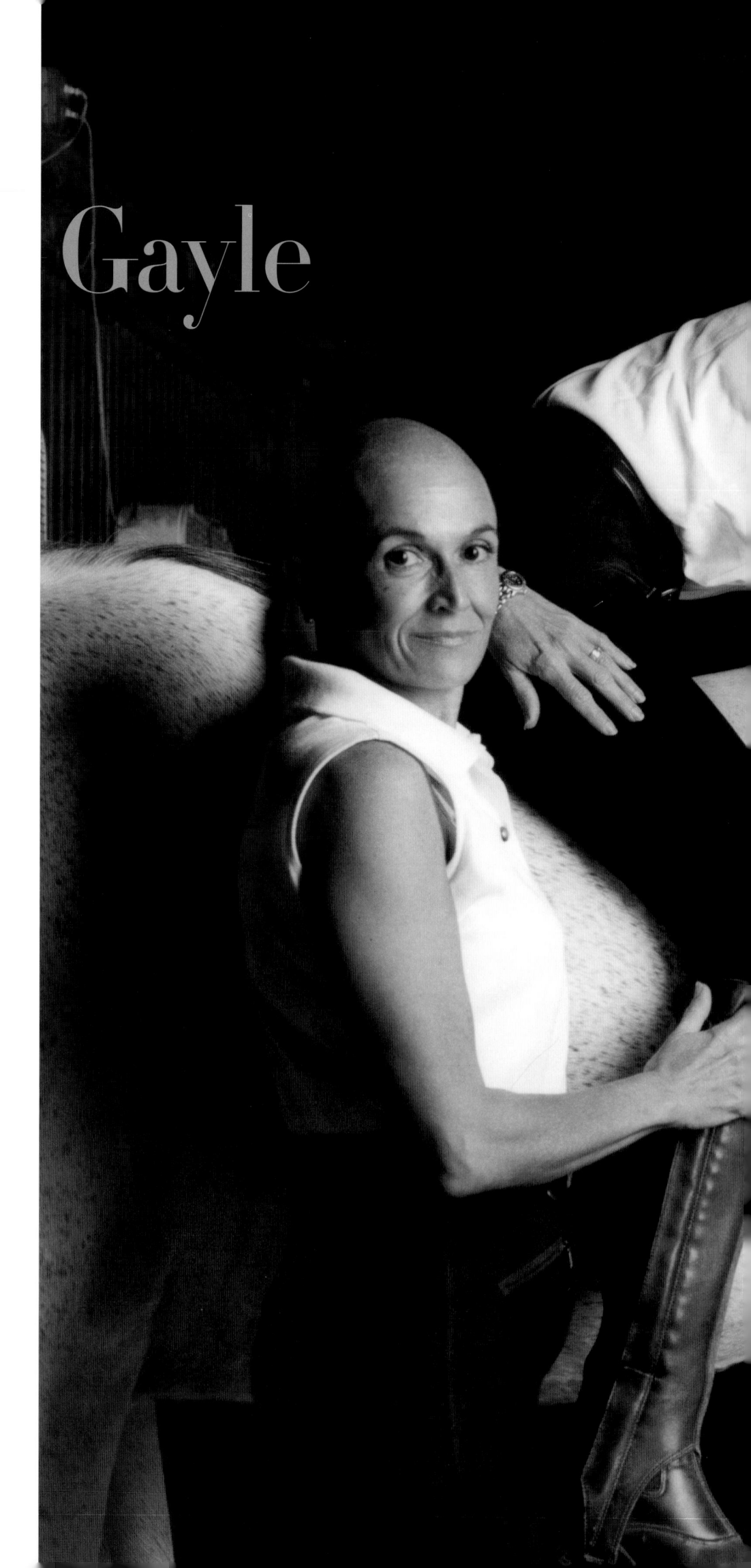

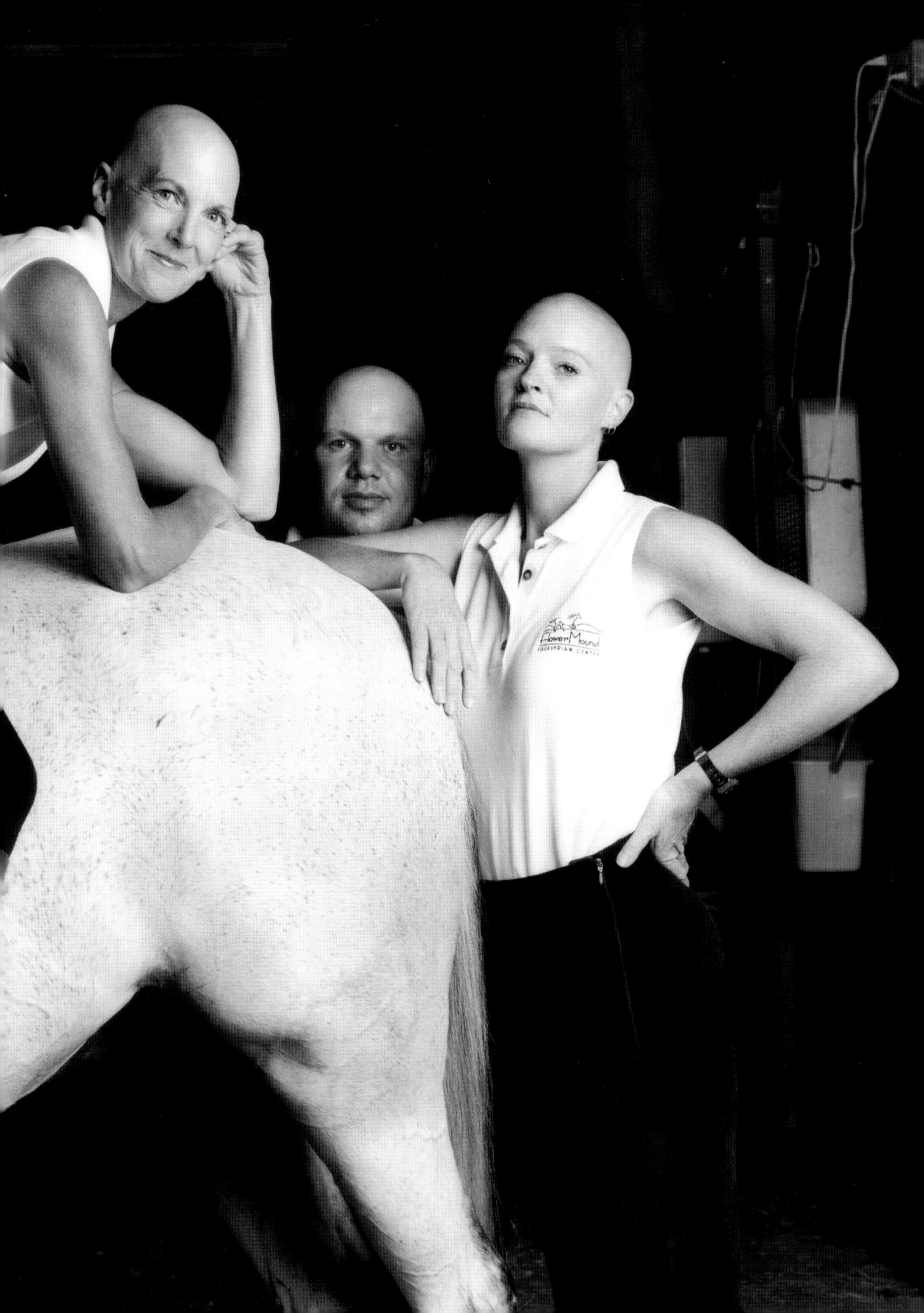

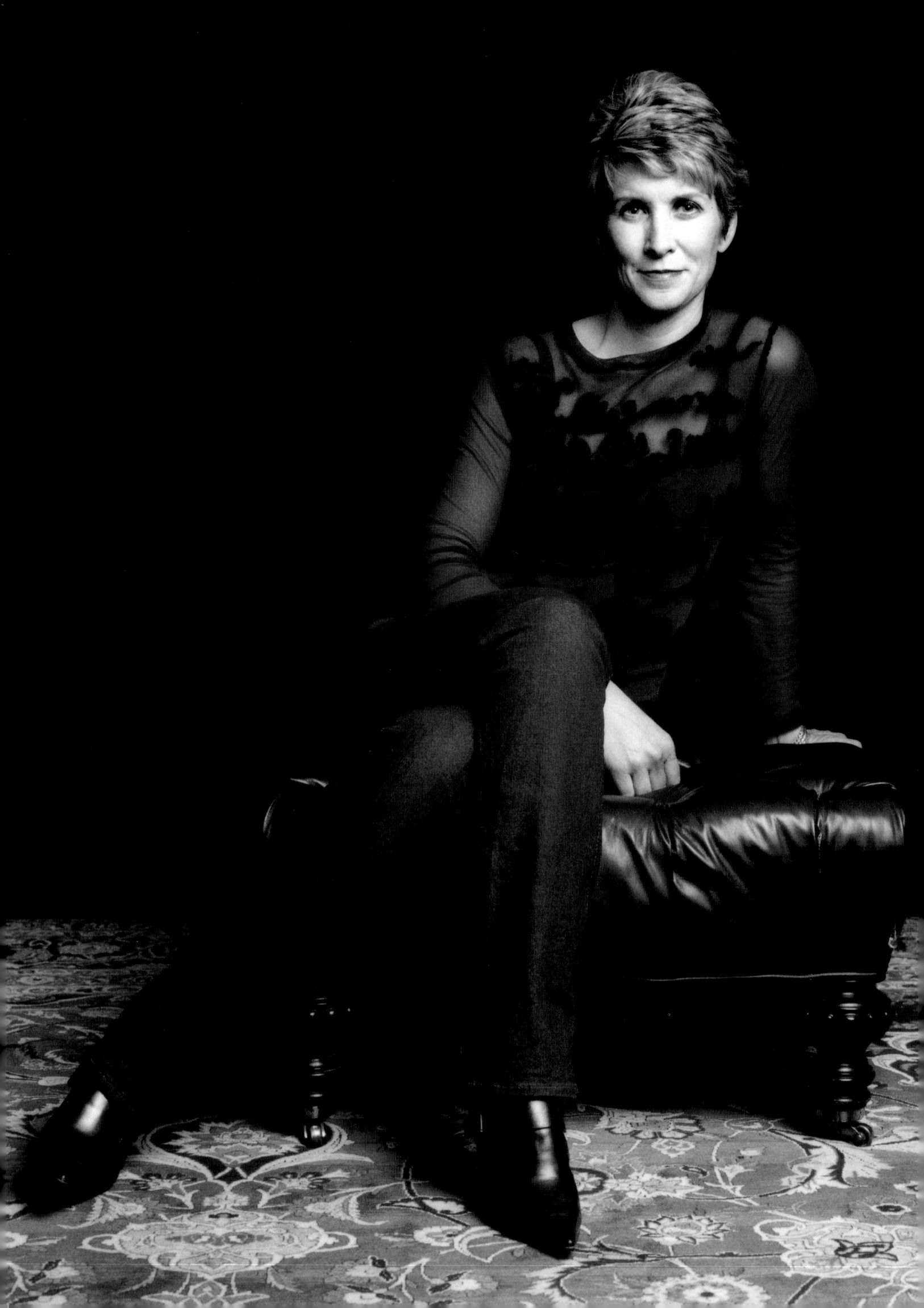

Laura

The mayor of Dallas, Texas, Laura Miller says her "world was badly tilted" after she was diagnosed with breast cancer at the age of thirty-nine. She says one part of her experience that really struck her was a feeling of loneliness in the midst of others who were going about their daily lives, despite the fact that her husband did his best to provide her with a supportive safety net.

"People always ask me how I stay so calm and cool in my job, through one 'crisis' after another," she says. "Easy. I survived cancer. My husband and kids are healthy. The rest is just noise."

Elizabeth

Elizabeth Merritt was named after her grandmother, who died of breast cancer. Today, at eighty-nine, she is a grandmother herself—and a survivor. A retired widow, she lives in her own apartment in a retirement community in Taos, New Mexico. Her roommate is a budgie bird named Crocodile Dundee. "I call this my Shangri-La," she says.

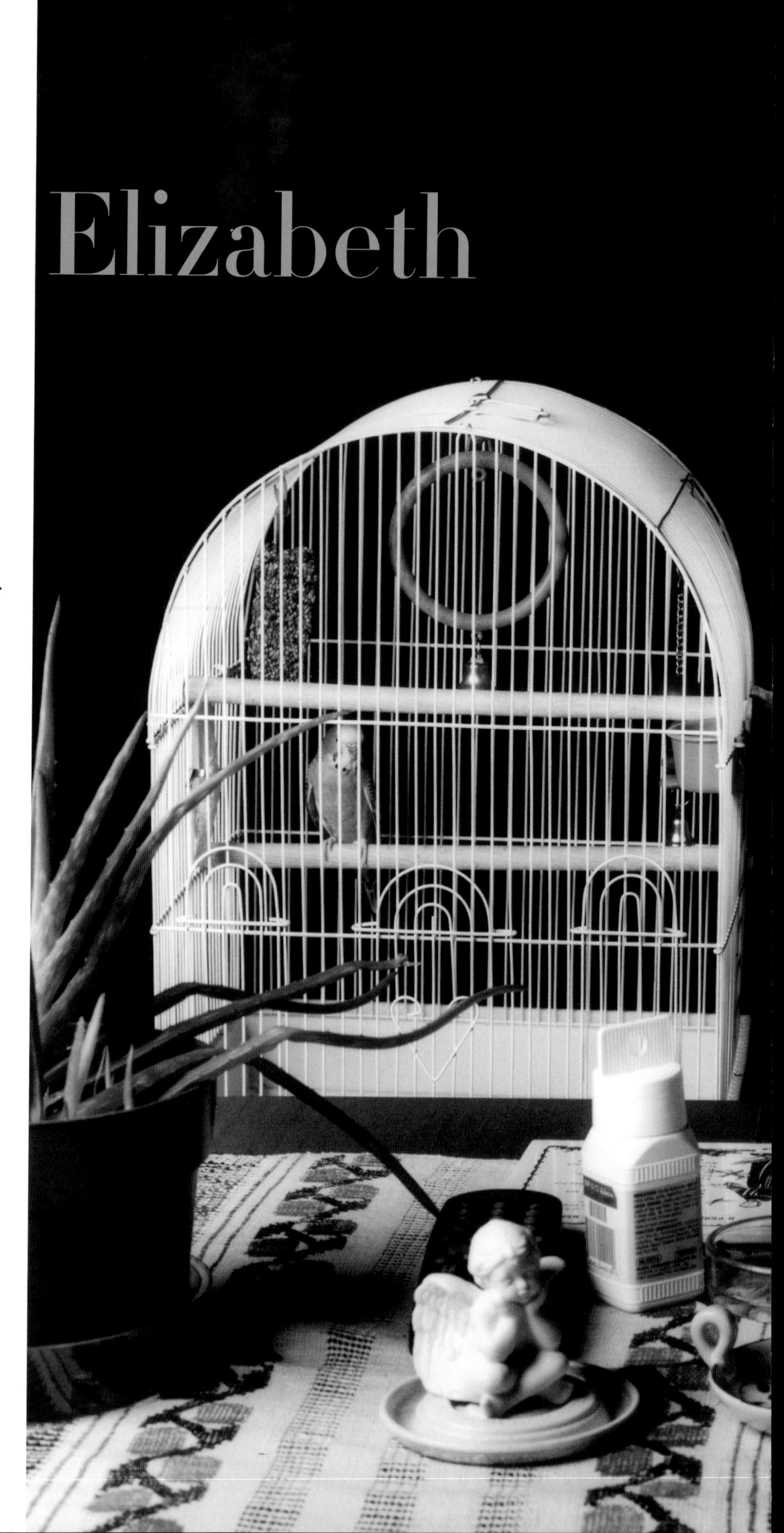

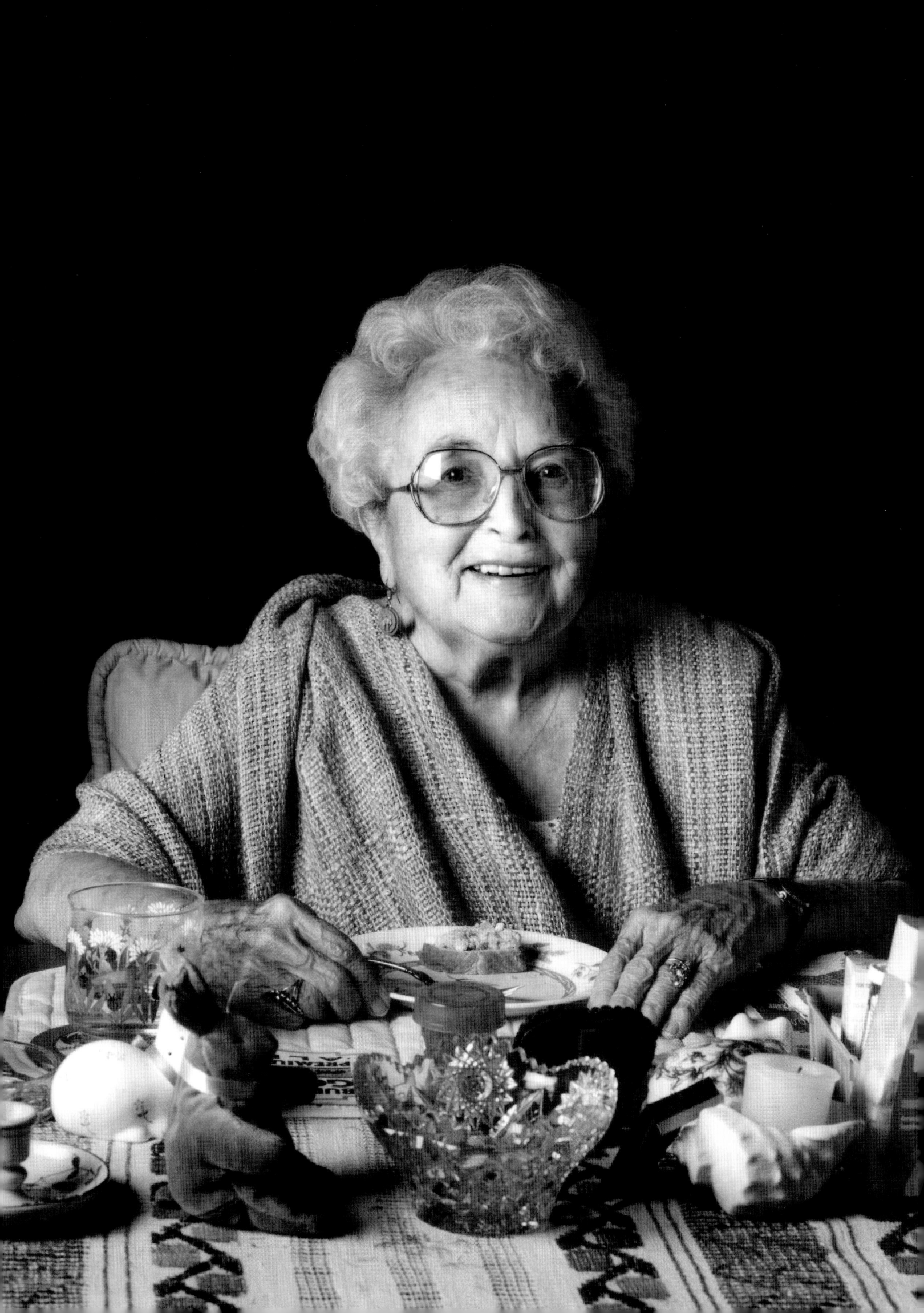

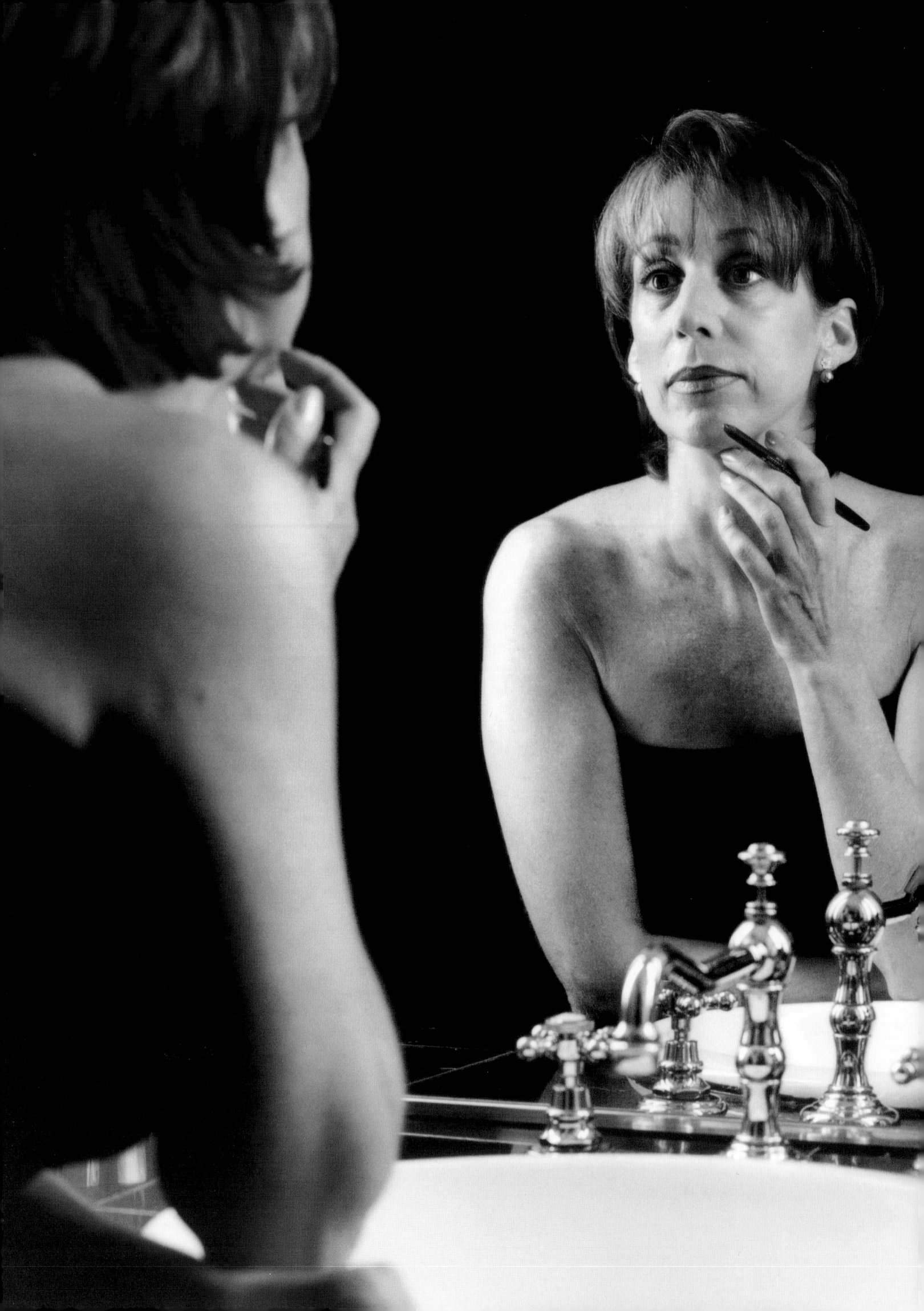

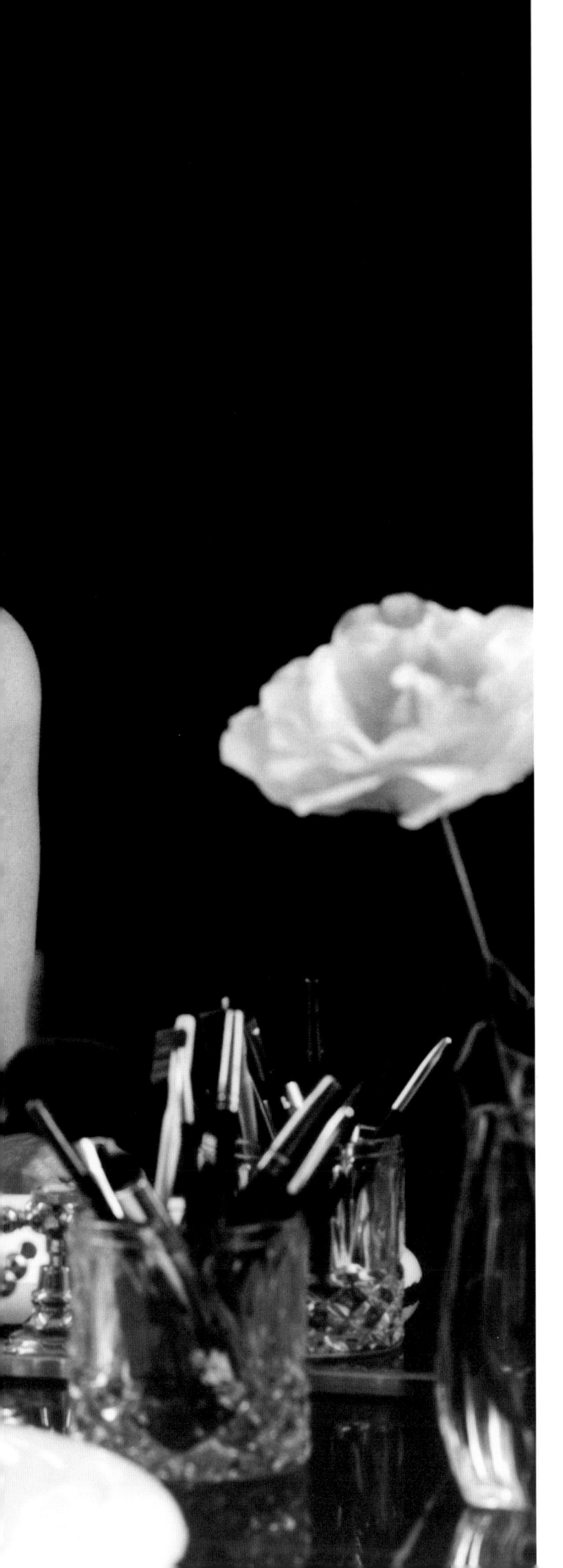

Jane

When Jane E. Pollock was diagnosed with breast cancer in 1993 at the age of forty-five, she was a successful makeup artist in addition to being a wife and busy mother of three children. During her treatment, she began using her makeup talents to assist fellow patients, adding color to their pale skin and the areas where their eyebrows and eyelashes once were. A Fox News affiliate in her hometown of Houston caught wind of the story, and tapes of the station's feature on Jane continue to circulate, inspiring others with her story and educating men and women about the issues surrounding cancer treatment. "This isn't just about makeup," she says. "It's sharing the experience. It's one way I can give back and continue to help."

Today Jane and her husband spend most of their time at their second residence on the beach in Coronado, California, "making life as stress-free as possible." She continues to counsel women with breast cancer.

Bitsy

"The day I was diagnosed with breast cancer, my bubble burst," says Bitsy Proler. Now, at age seventy, this wife, mother, grandmother, and author is making new bubbles. Her cancer experience inspired her to tap into her spiritual side, and today she embraces writing, painting, and astrology as outlets for her new appreciation for life.

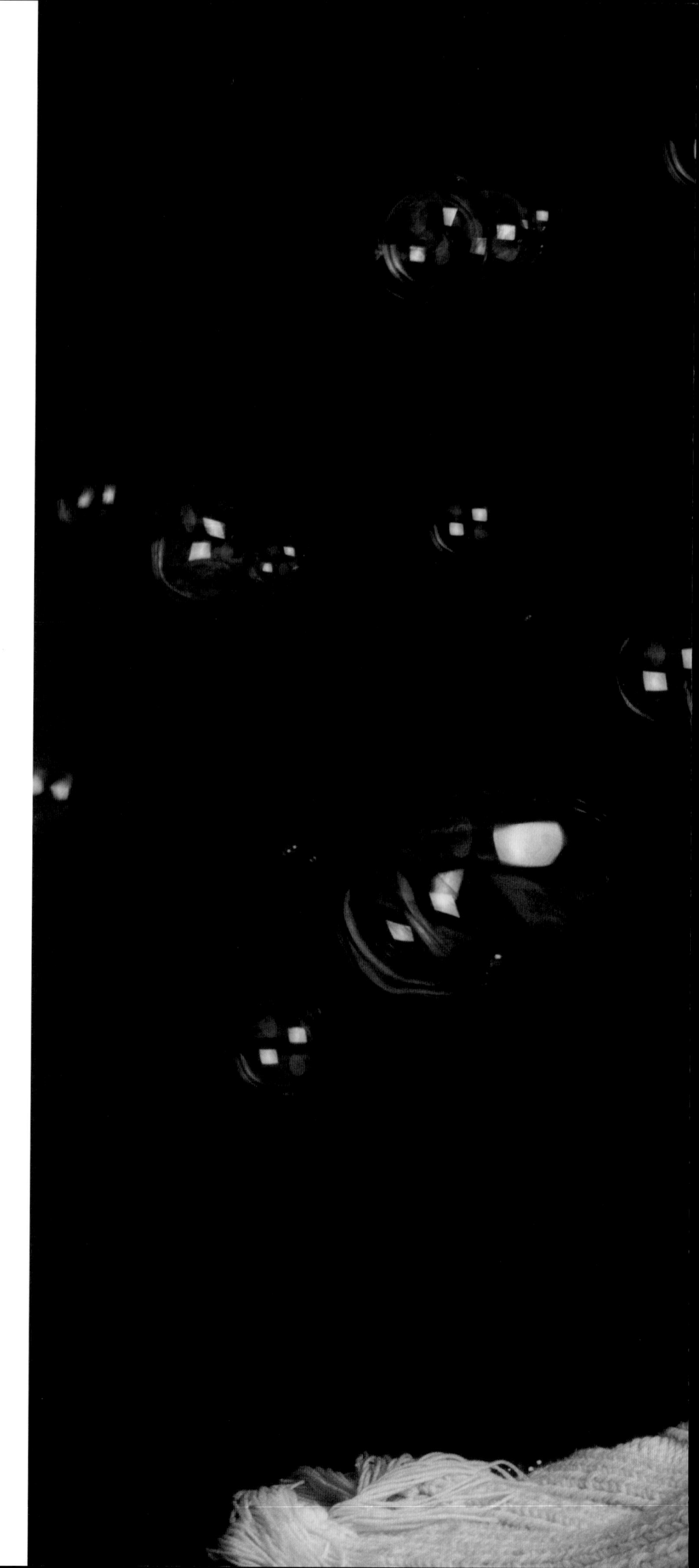

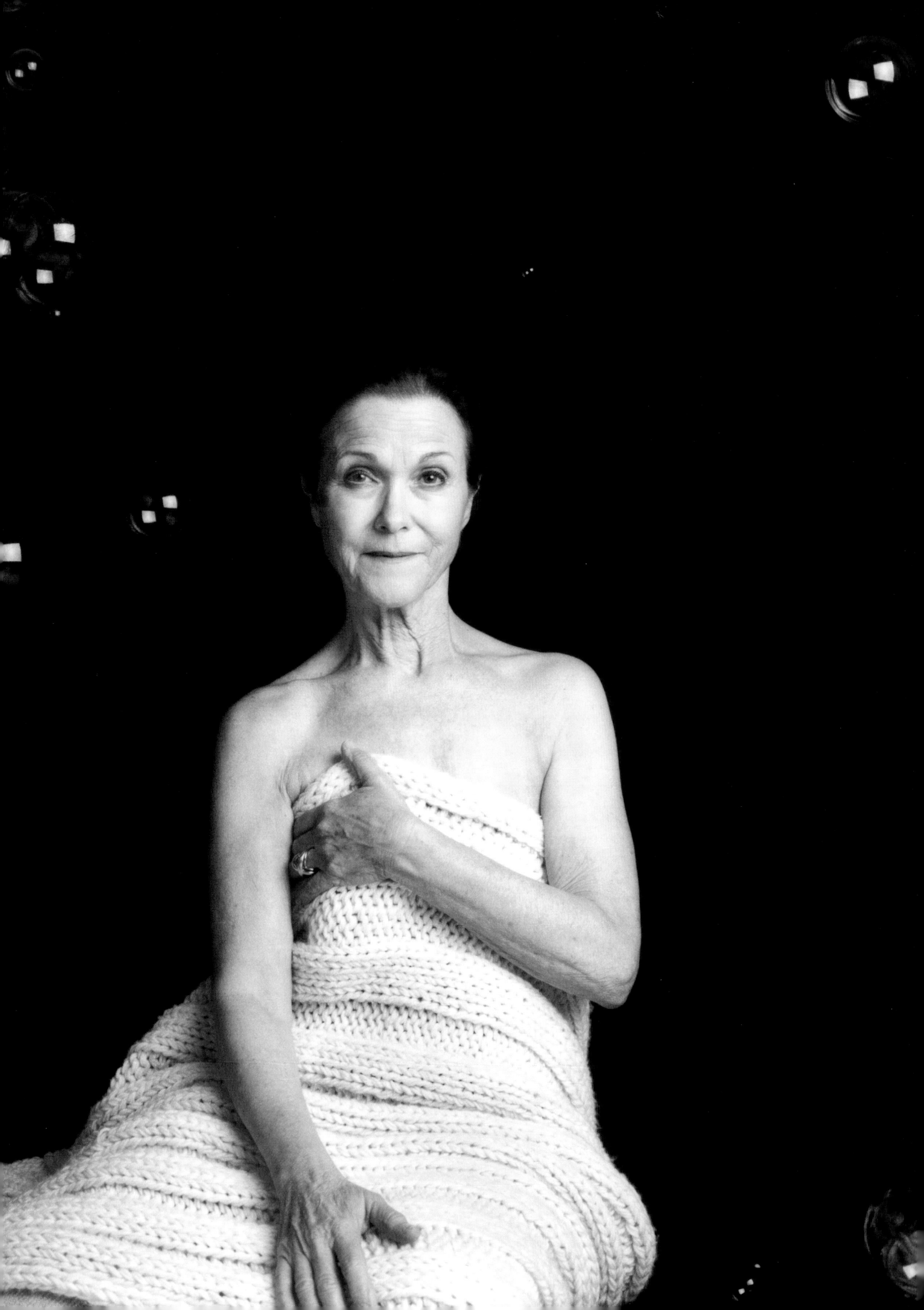

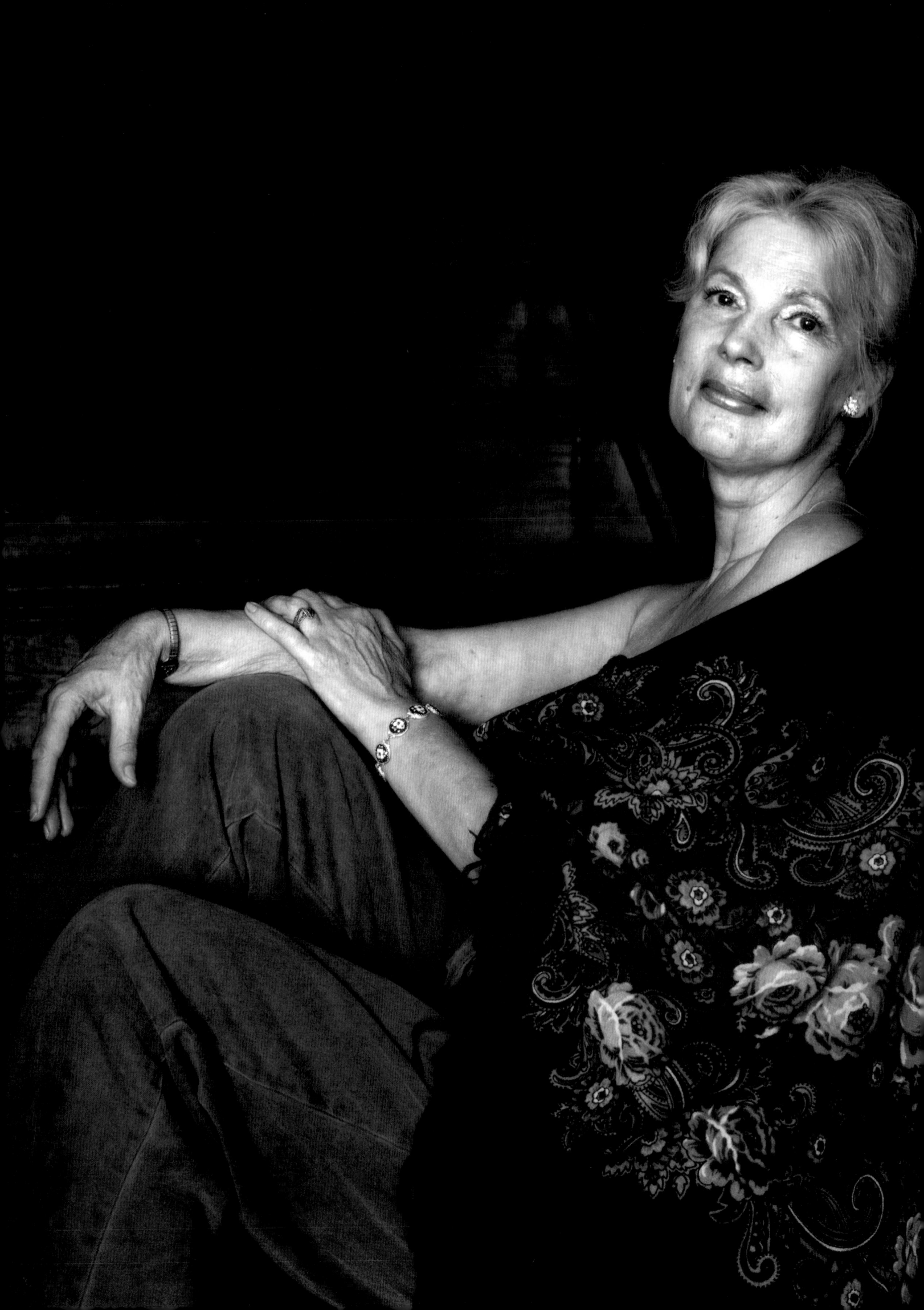

Lyudmila

A native of Russia who now lives outside of Boston with her family, Lyudmila Rudyakov was diagnosed with breast cancer in 1999. She says that simply being in the United States helped to calm her fears about the disease. "Here I will be treated the best way," she says.

Ann and Eugenia

Ann Hudson (left) and Eugenia Lara met through Reach for Recovery, a Dallas, Texas, volunteer group established through the American Cancer Society. They identified with each other's experiences with breast cancer, and became fast friends. "When in Dallas, we shared those years together once a week with a martini and lunch," Eugenia says.

Today, the women have moved from the Dallas area to smaller Texas towns fifty miles apart, but they continue to see and support each other on a regular basis. A native of Mexico, Eugenia has concentrated her volunteer efforts toward helping Hispanic women, translating brochures and videos about chemotherapy into Spanish.

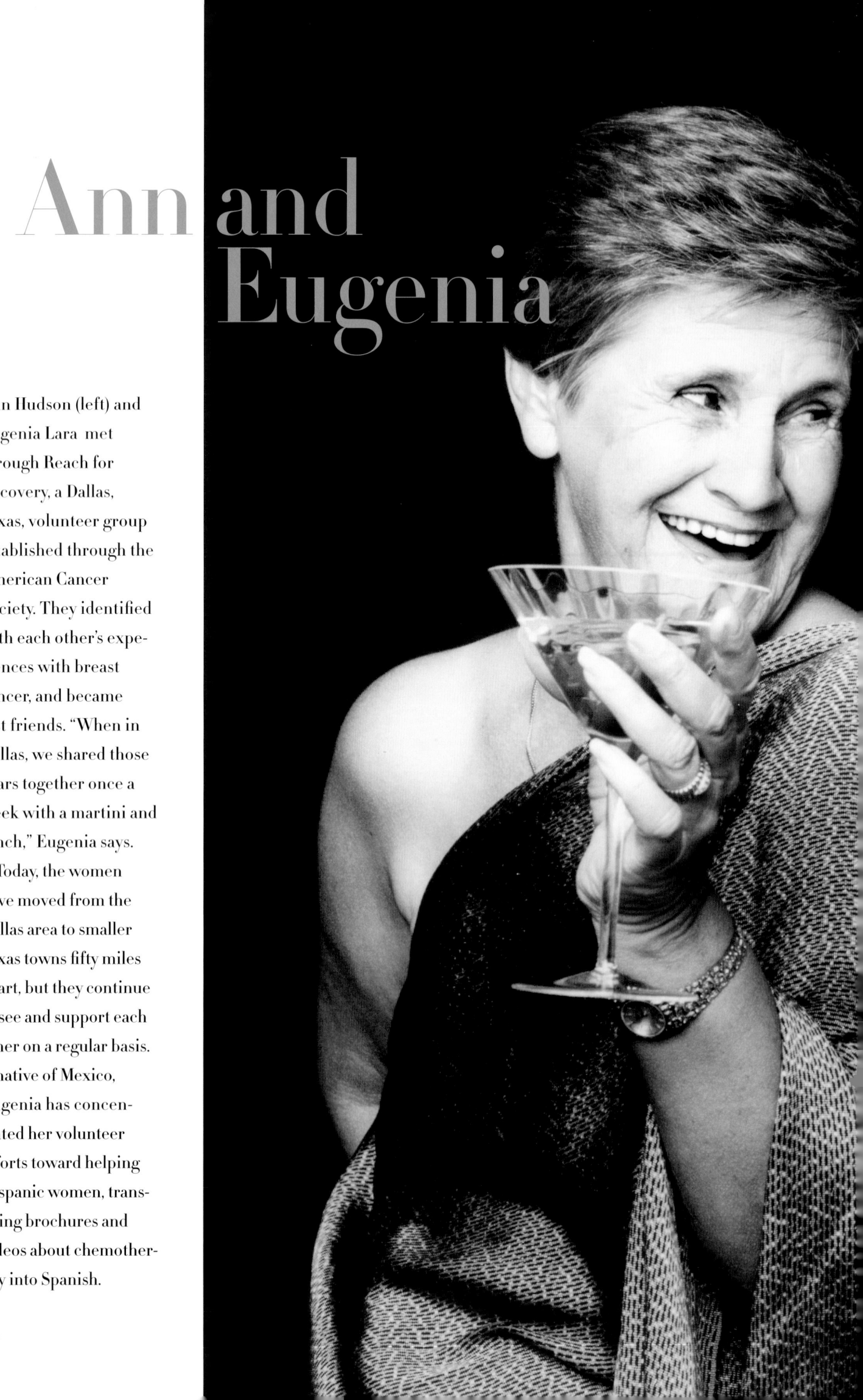

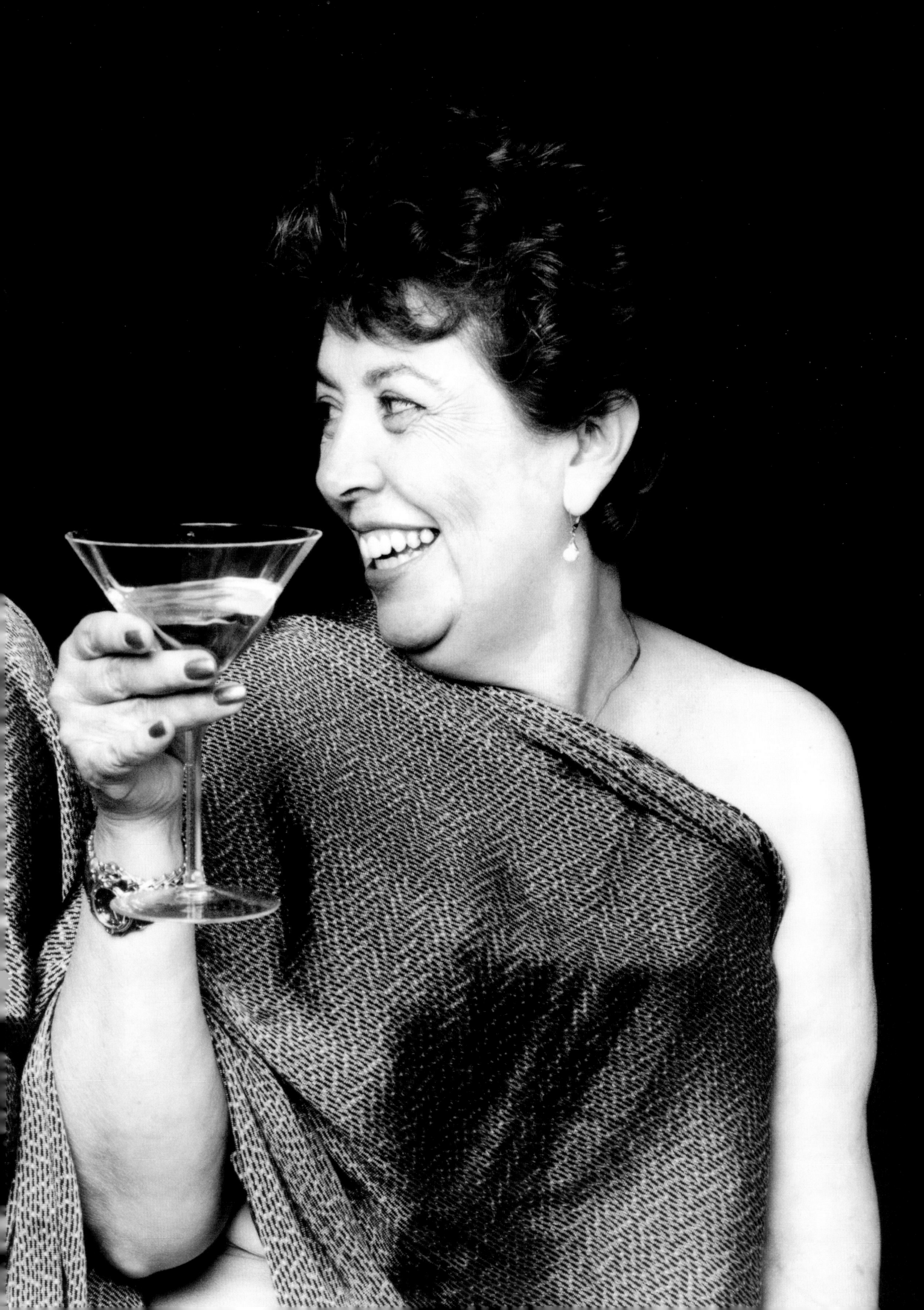

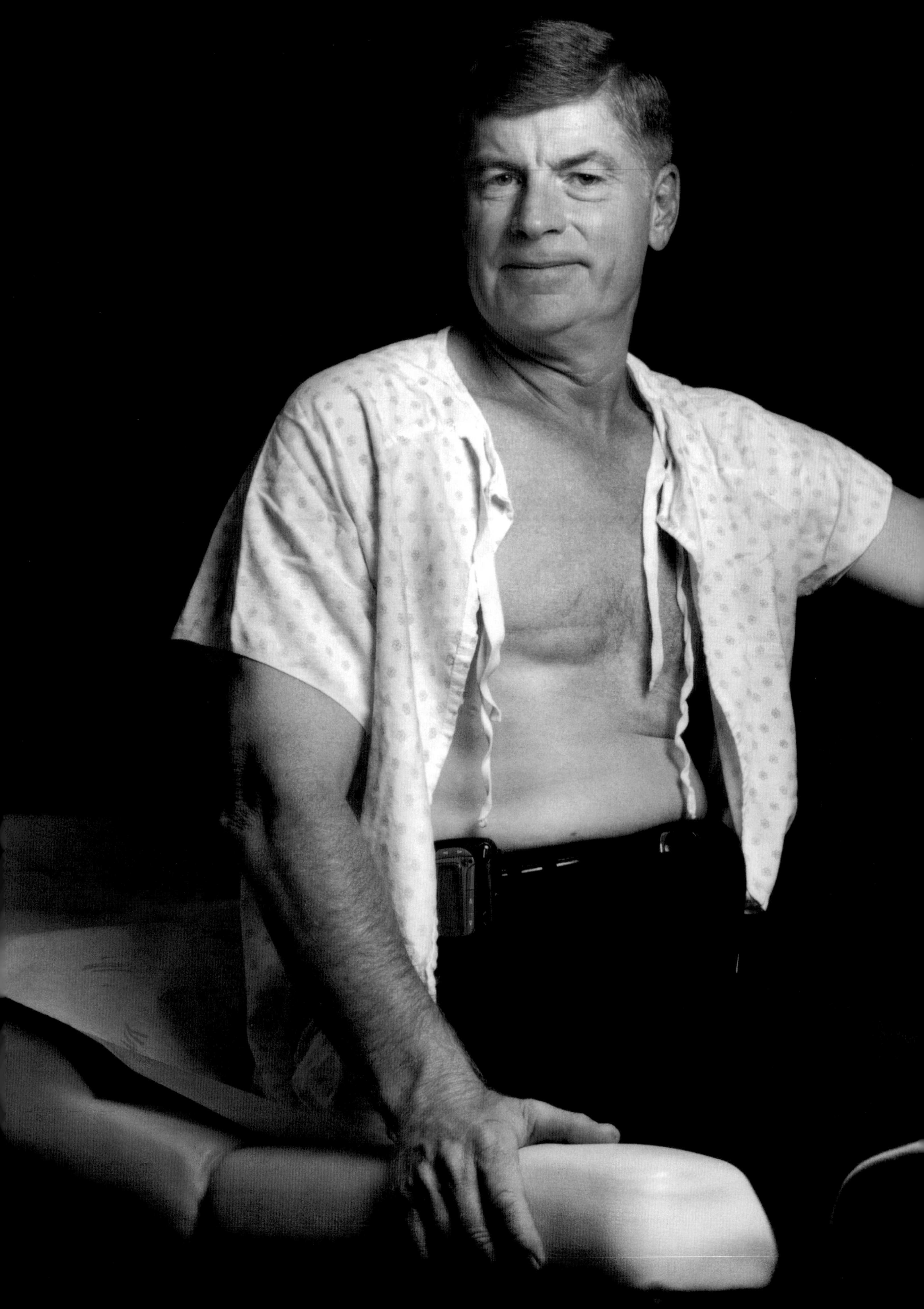

Alan

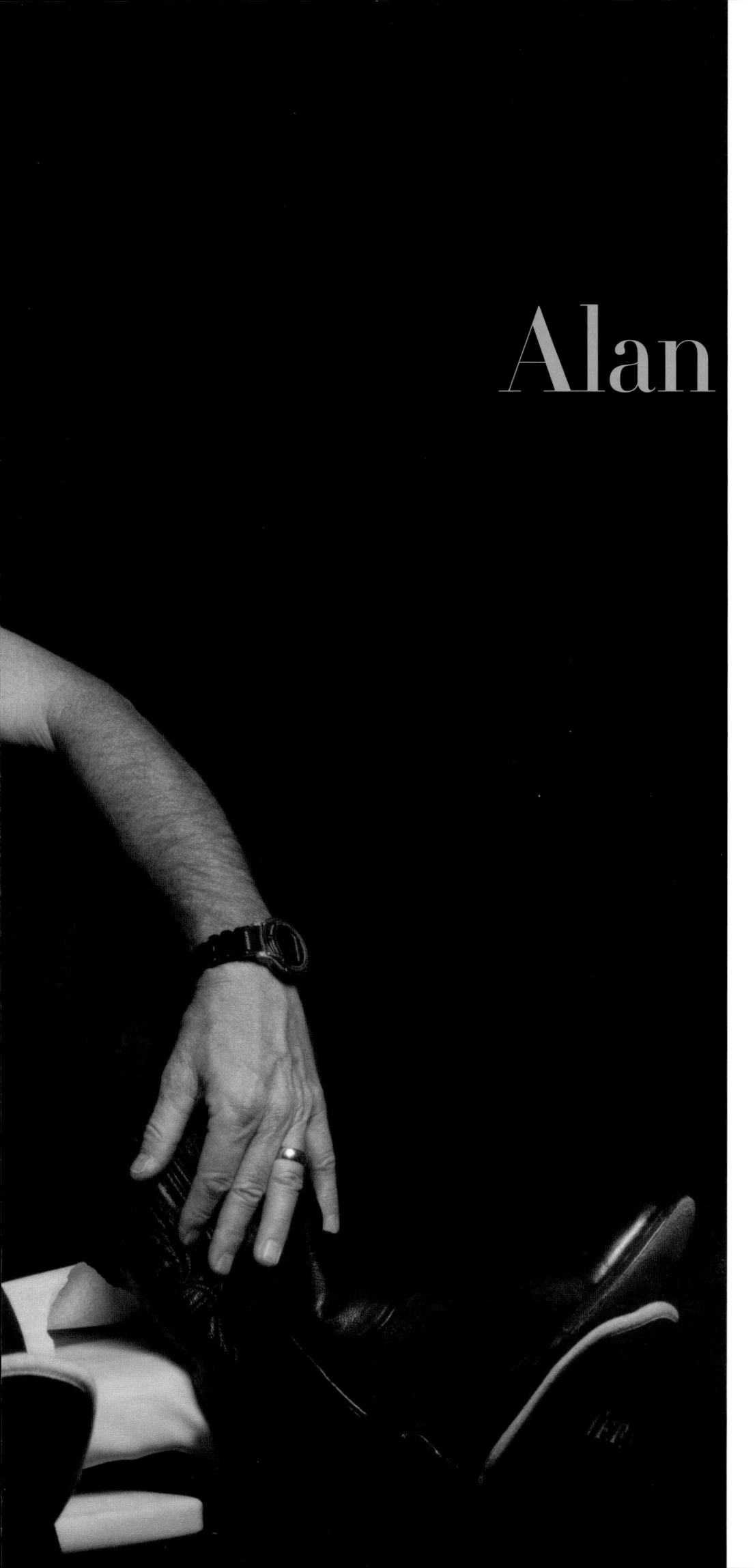

In his Fort Worth, Texas, obstetrics and gynecology practice, Dr. Alan Johns provides care for women dealing with cancer on a daily basis. But when he found himself on the flipside of the doctor/patient relationship in 1998, he felt the effect beyond his personal life—as a husband and father—and into his professional one. "I never really thought about when one of my patients were actually diagnosed. I just went through the process with them," he says. "Now my patients elect to use me as their physician."

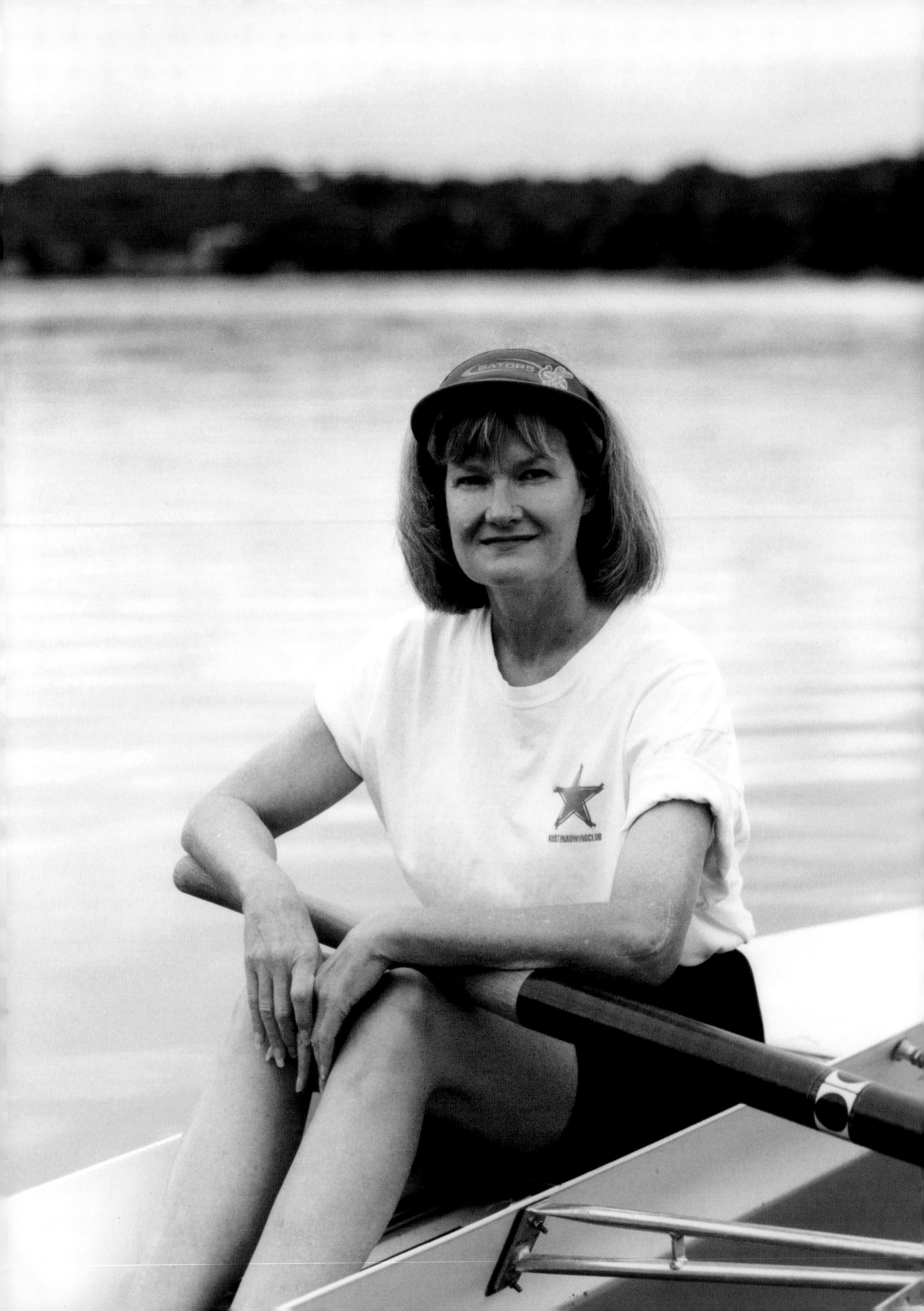
GATORS
AUSTINROWINGCLUB

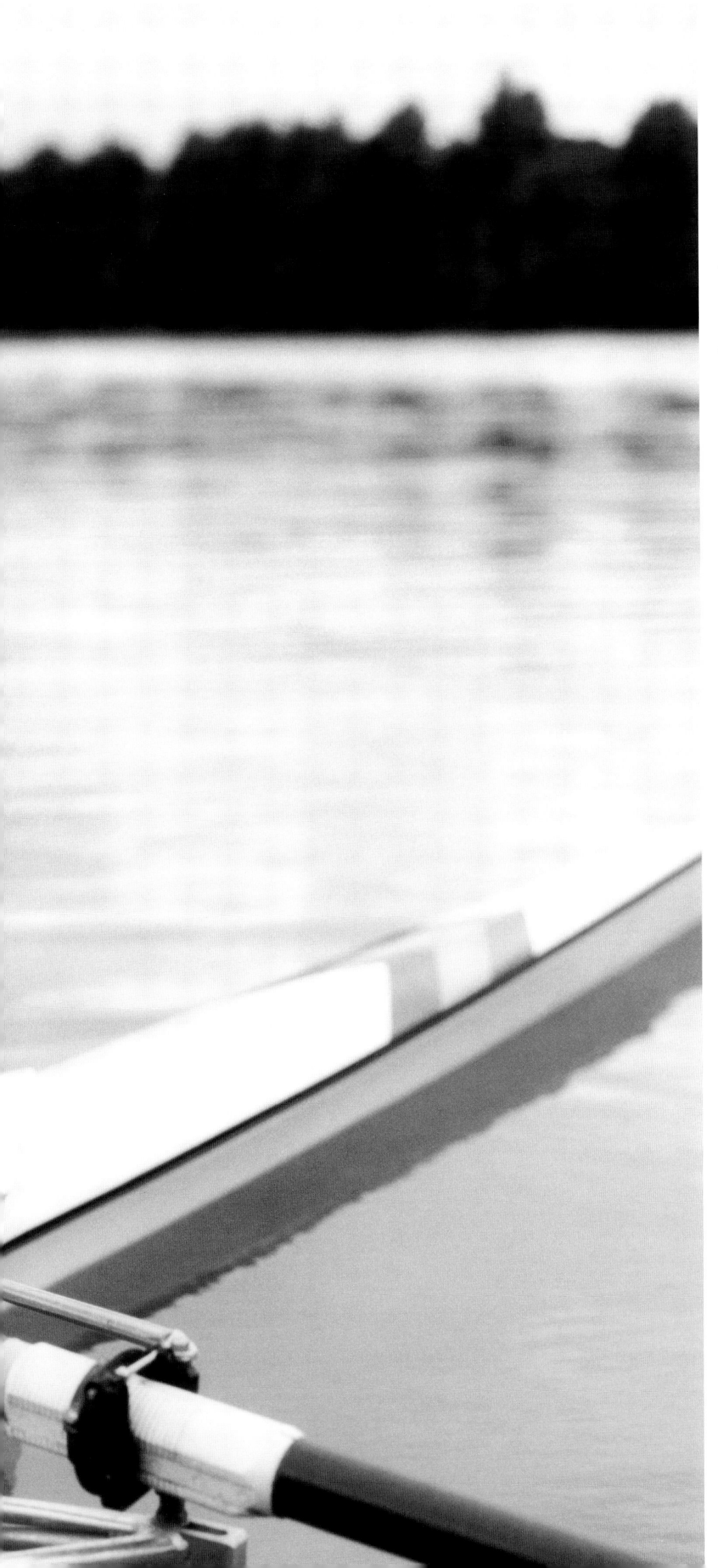

Peggy

The director of the Texas Department of Mental Health and Retardation, Peggy Perry was a self-described workaholic before she was diagnosed with breast cancer seven years ago. Yet it was not her work, but her love for rowing with a local crew team that ultimately helped her to prepare for the challenges she faced with her mastectomy and lymphodema. As it turned out, some of the other women in her rowing club were breast cancer survivors, and they served as a ready-made support system for Peggy as she worked to face those challenges on her own. Touched by the bond she formed with her teammates, Peggy now helps to counsel others facing the disease.

Christine

A single mother and one of only two women on the 117-man Texas Rangers, Christine Nix is no stranger to confronting challenges on a daily basis. So it's only fitting that when she was being treated for breast cancer, her oncology team named her "Cancer Hero of the Year." After her second bout with the disease, Christine decided to throw her wig away. "I'm sick, not flawed," she says. "I was going to wage my one-person war against society's unspoken rule of what identifies us: appearance."

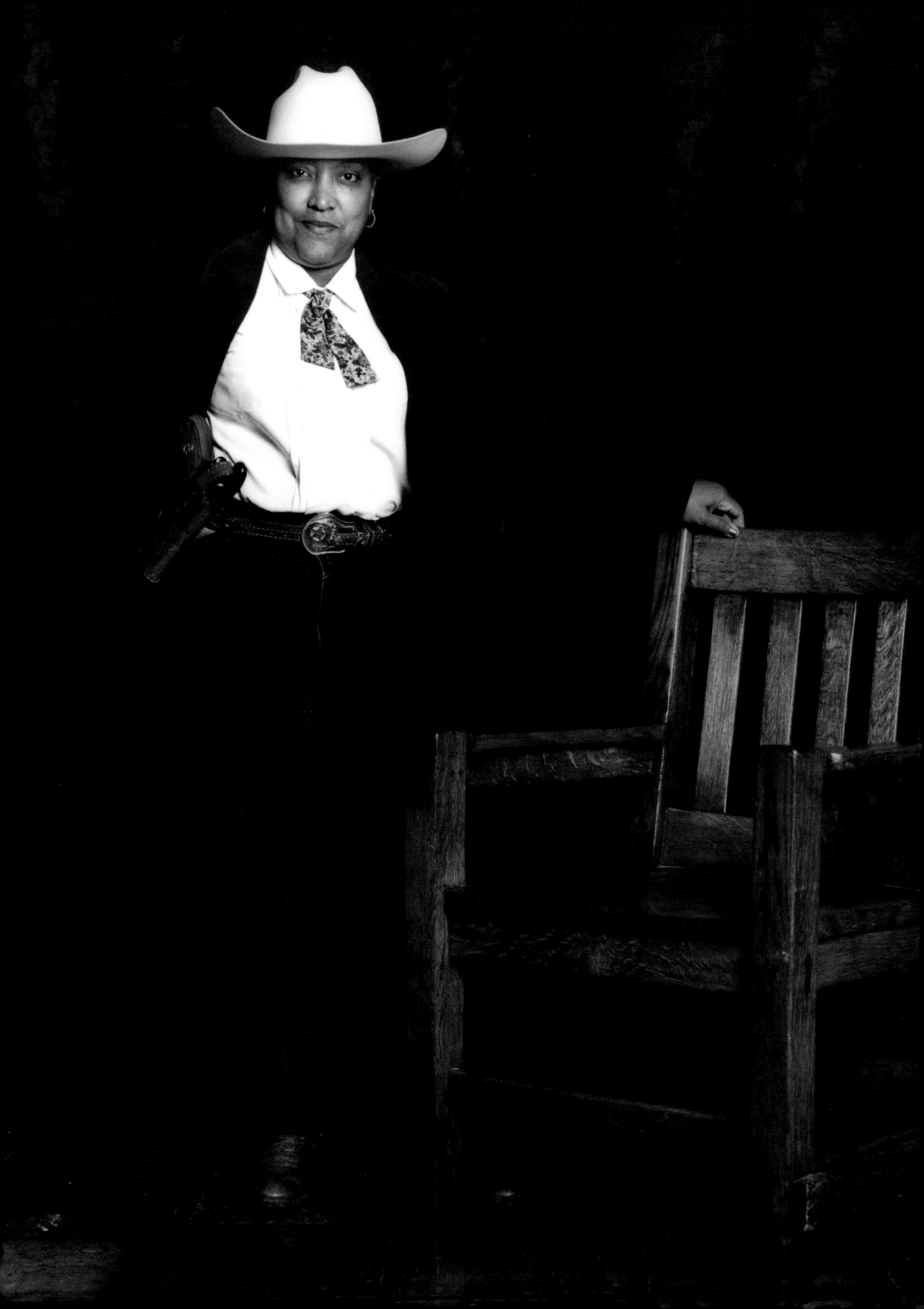

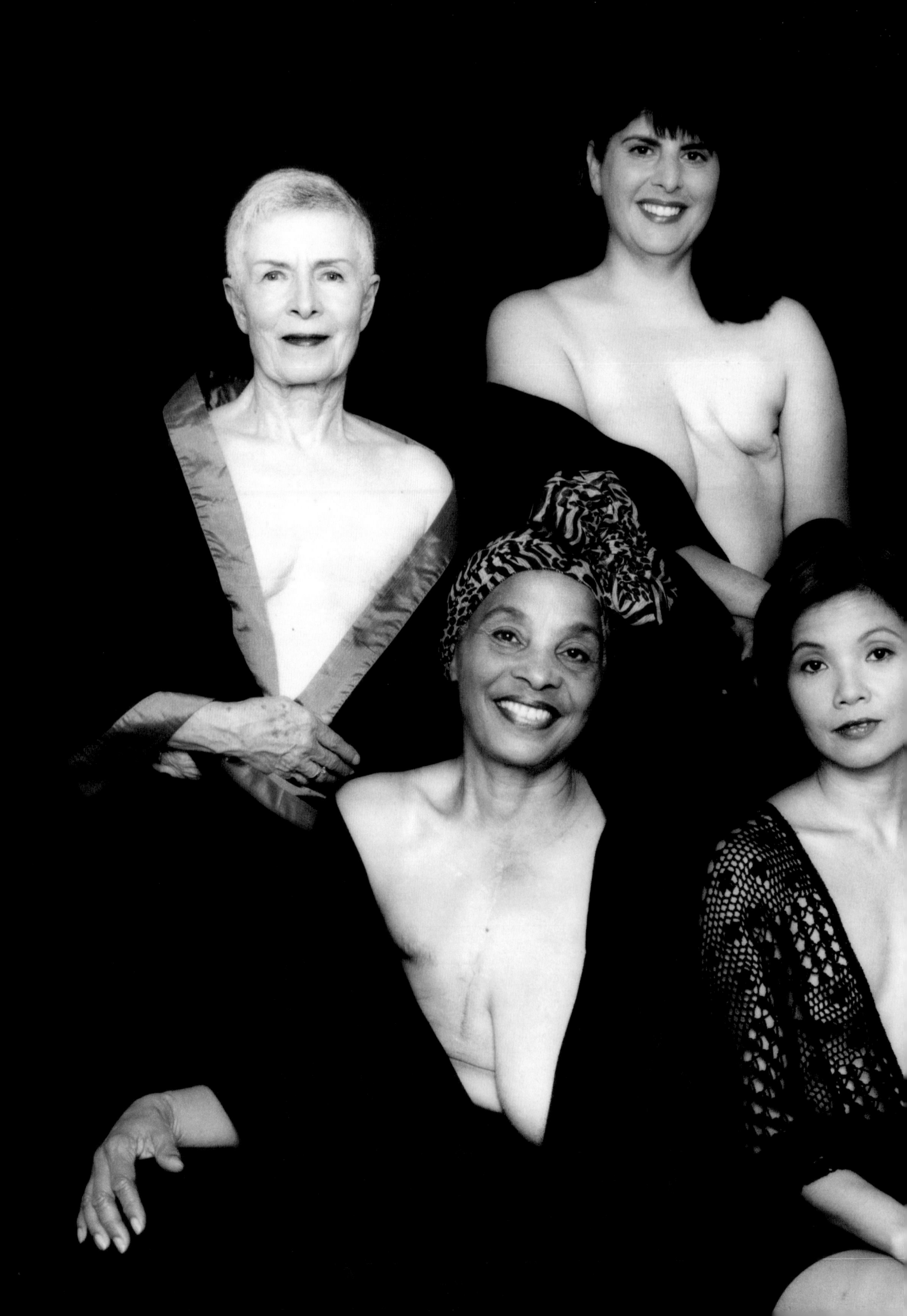

Lois, Shakay, Gloria, Pearl, Elena, and Lisa

I first met this very special group of survivors at a photo shoot featuring women who had had mastectomies for the now-defunct *Rosie* magazine. All of them had the strength to bare their scars to help educate and inspire the magazine's readers nationwide, and each had a unique story to tell of her experience recovering from breast cancer.

Top row, from left:
Lois Tschetter Hjelmstad (also on page 119), Shakay J. Kizirian, Gloria Aponte;
Front row, from left:
Pearl Griffith-Eccles, Elena Comendador, Lisa Opperman

Darrell

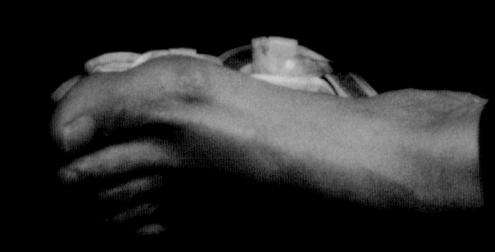

Believe it or not, Darrell Kirkland has been married to a man named Daryl for more than thirty-five years. She distinguishes the spelling of their names by pointing out that hers has two R's and two L's and his doesn't. "Before breast cancer," she jokes, "I used to have two of everything."

Not only did Darrell decline reconstruction when a cancerous lump was discovered in one breast, but she insisted that both breasts be removed at that time. Her decision was influenced by personal experiences working with terminally ill hospice patients, though she admits her oncologist was dumbfounded by her aggressive stance. "Cancer is simply a disease you pass through," she insists.

Darrell has experience in the matter beyond her own, having lost a nephew and a father to cancer. She is pictured here with her granddaughter Berit, the first of her three grandchildren. "My grandchildren are the best reasons for my existence," she says. "My photo says everything, because it is the happiest time of my life."

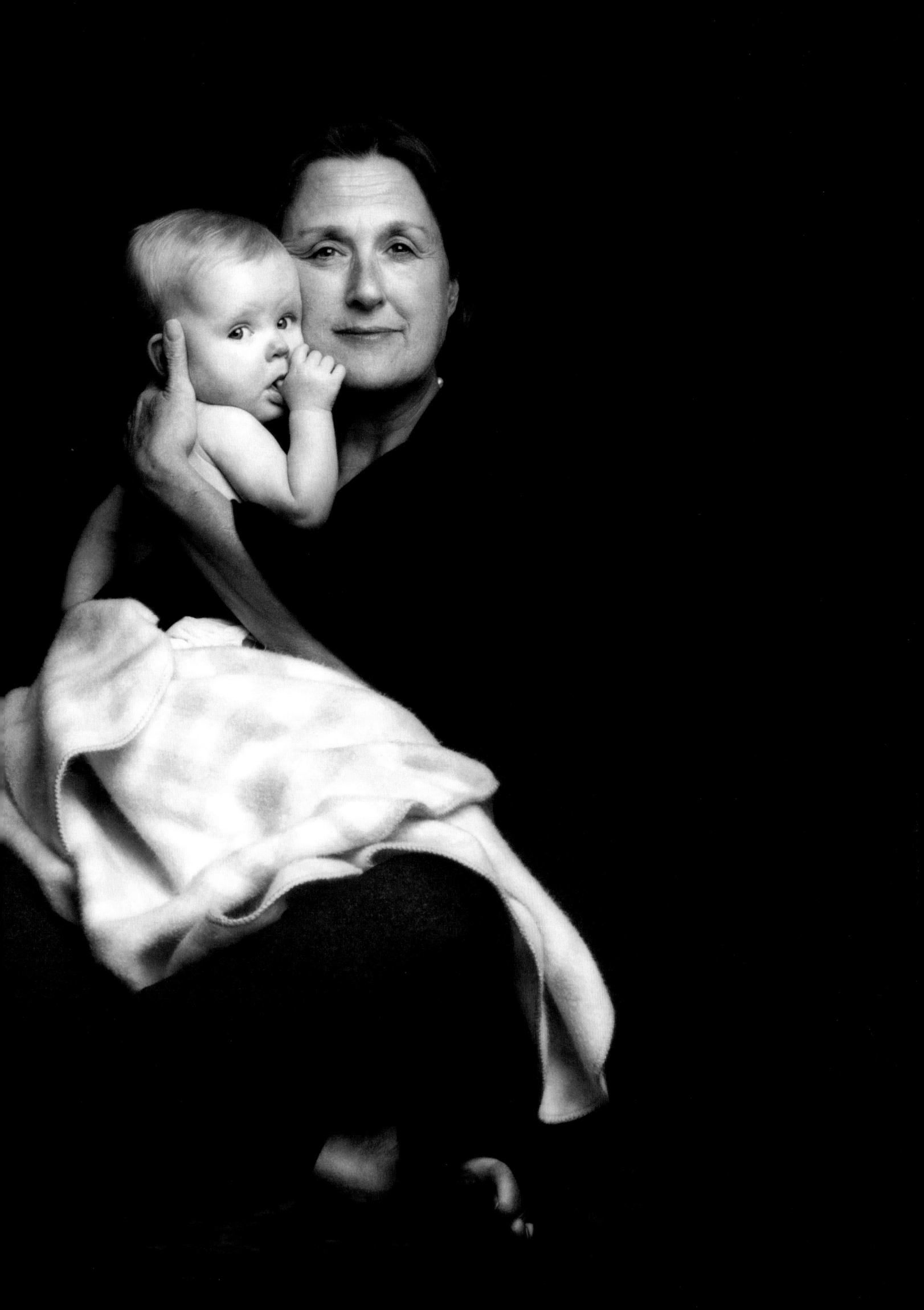

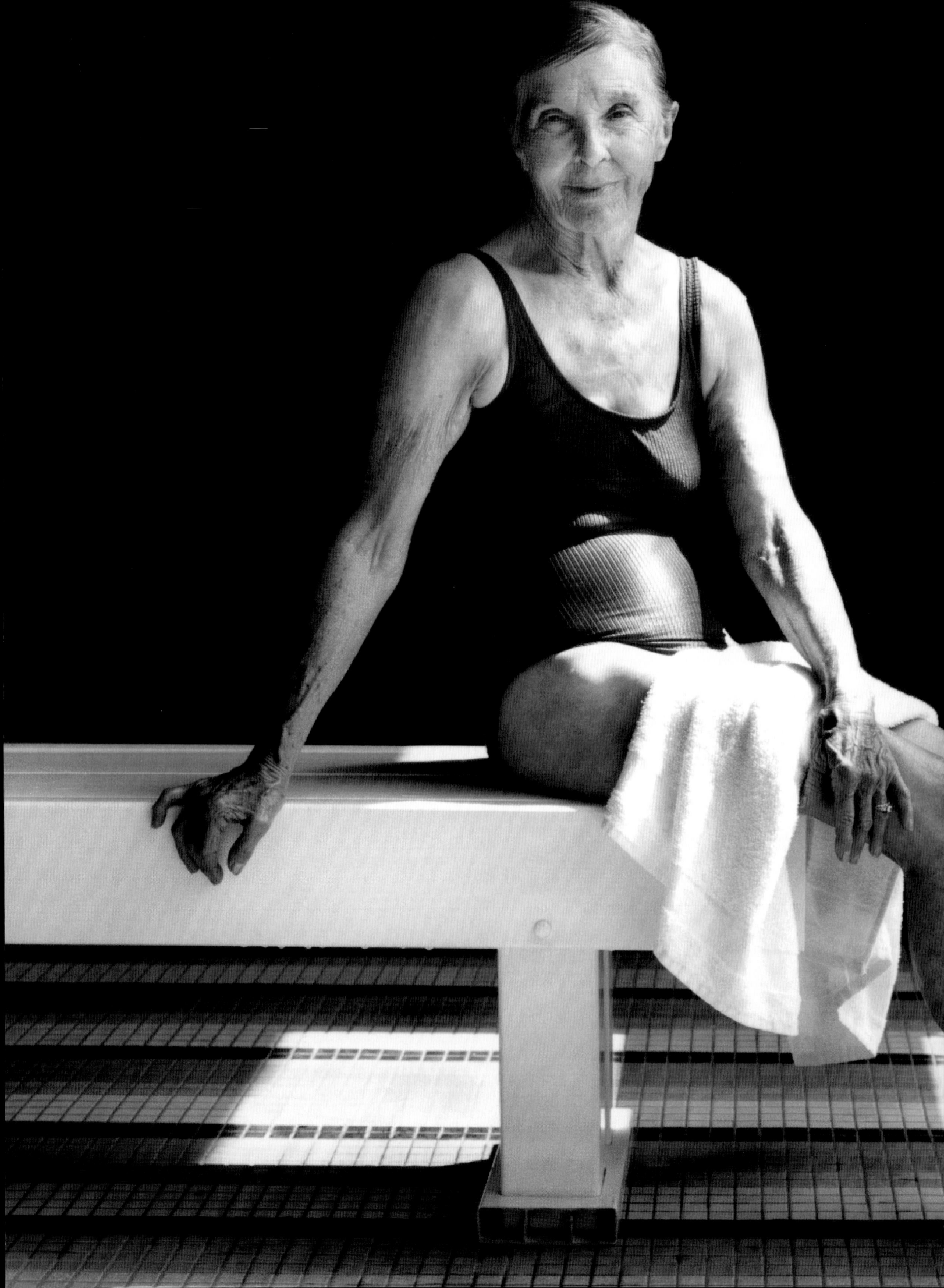

Fran

A retired pilot, Fran Shelton has substituted swimming for flying. At eighty-three, ten years after her cancer diagnosis, she may be better suited for the ground, but she still holds dear her years spent in the clouds. Fran was a longtime member of Dallas's Red Bird Chapter of the '99ers women flyers organization. This group of adventuresome women would fly from Texas to Oklahoma just to have lunch with friends. "We were never dull!"

Julie and Judith

Twins, **Julie Ann Janaszak (left) and Judith Ann Olson** have experienced their lives together since day one, but they never imagined they'd experience breast cancer together, as well. Judith was diagnosed at age thirty, and though Julie has remained cancer-free, she devoted herself to being there for Judith.

"I recall speaking with Twin on the telephone about my plans to shave my head, and she wanting to do the same thing," Judith says. "Why would anyone *want* to do that, let alone actually *do* that? Days later, I suspected she shaved her head (even though I told her it wasn't necessary), but she never admitted it until the next time I saw her. We were in the middle of dining out and she pulled her wig off. I, in turn, pulled my wig off, and we hugged, cried, and laughed together. The entire restaurant joined in the experience by applauding us. This was a pivotal point in my recovery."

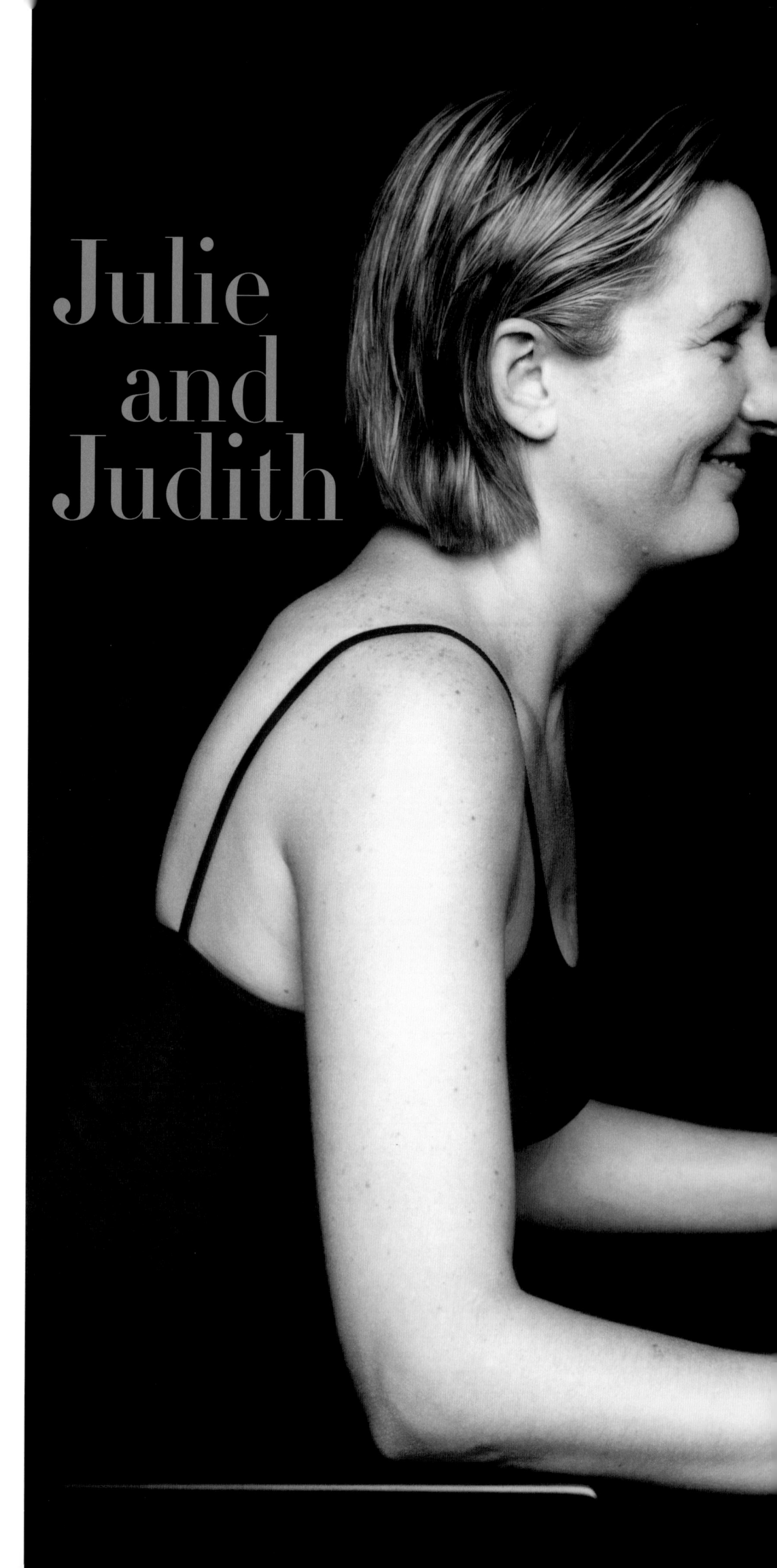

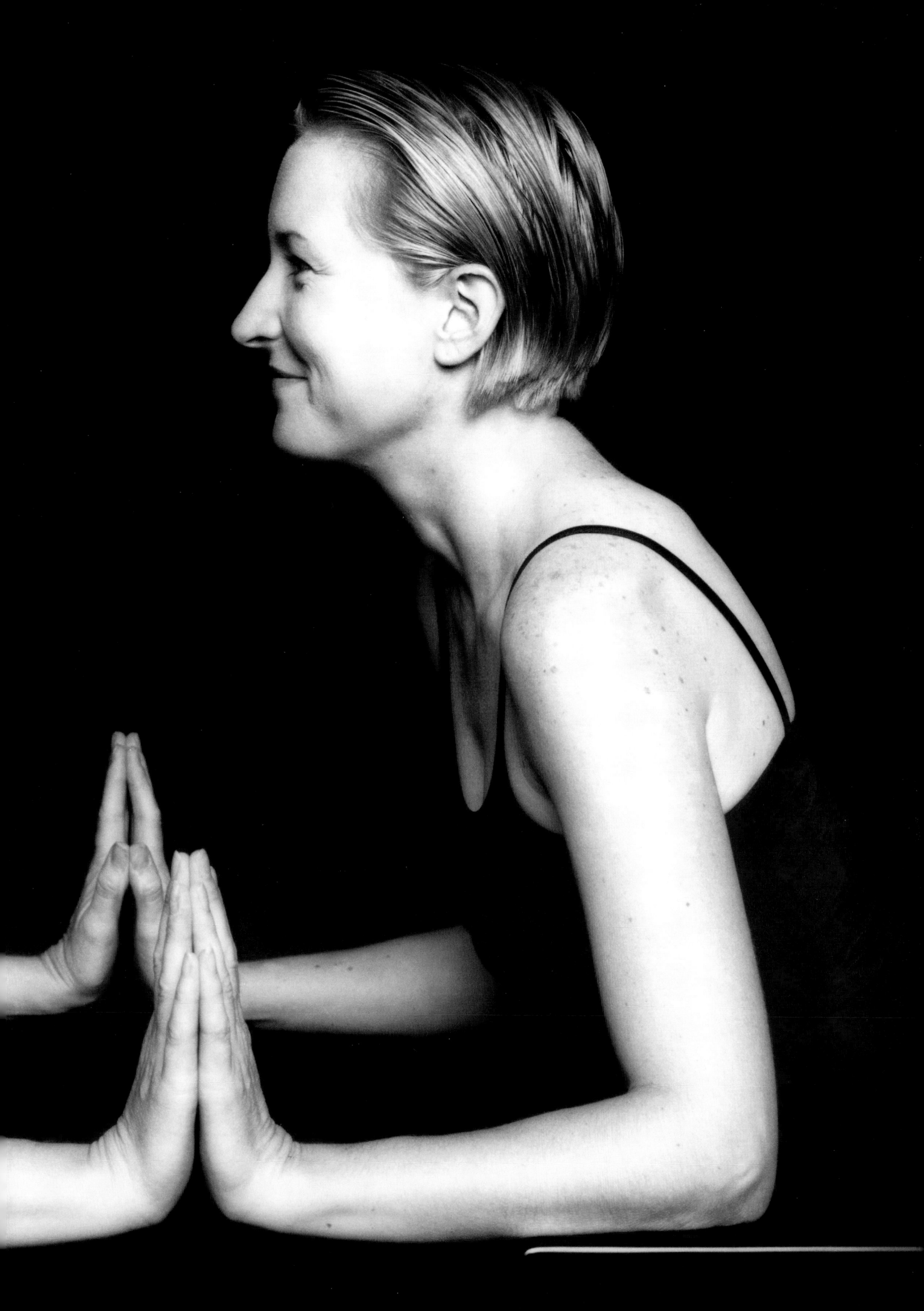

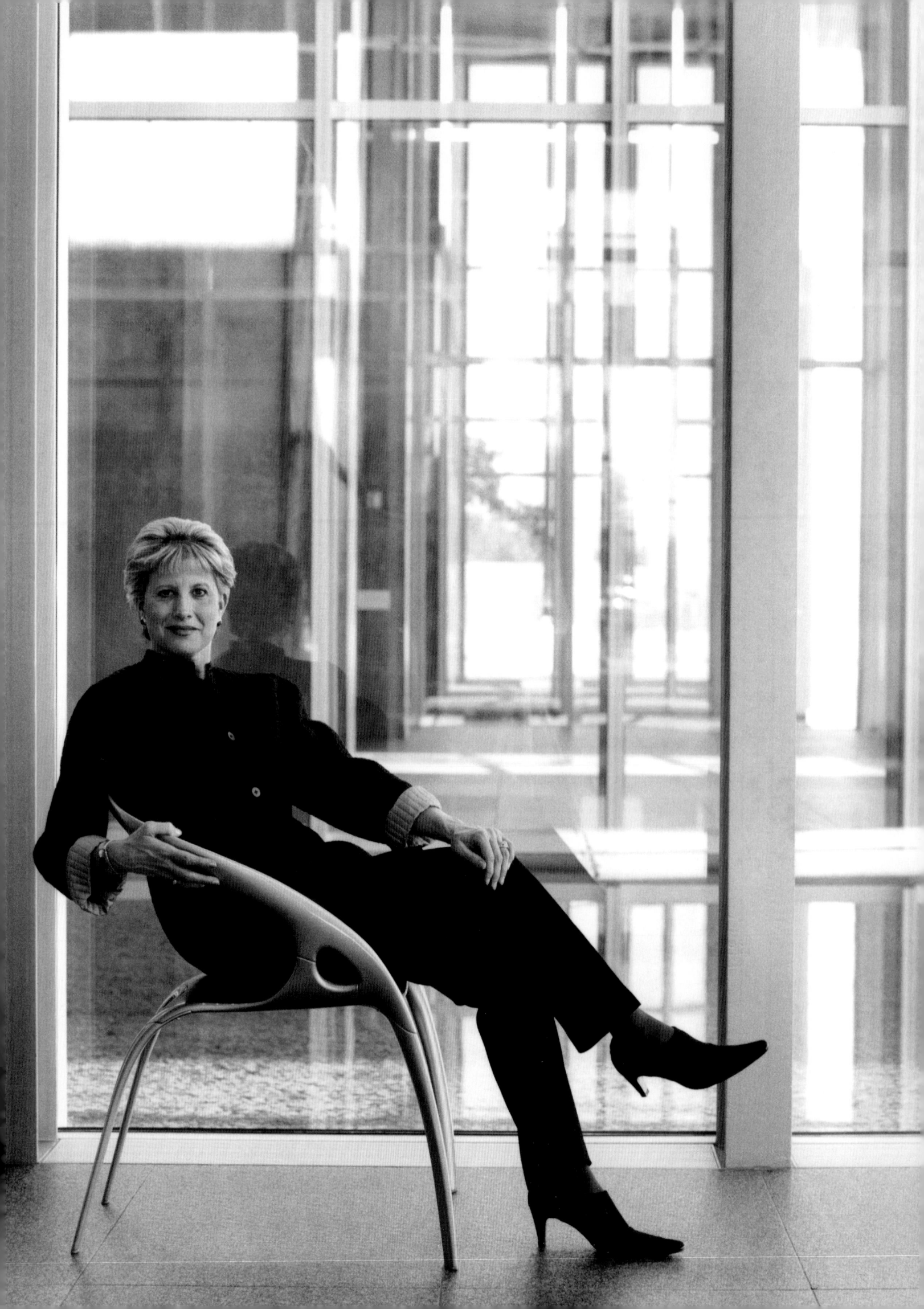

Joan

At the young age of thirty, Joan Katz awakened in an operating room to learn of her breast cancer diagnosis. "At that moment, all I could envision was a limited future. And I had no idea how wrong these feelings would turn out to be."

Although she has been diagnosed two more times since, she says that turning point in the hospital triggered in her a zest for life. She embraces even the smallest experiences with amazement. As a mother, she has treasured her time with her daughter, watching her learn to ride a bike, drive a car, and graduate high school. "I have gone snorkeling in the Caymans, kissed the Blarney Stone in Ireland, and led a conga line through the snow in Colorado. I have laughed, loved, dreamed, played, aged, shared, and tried to live each day to the fullest."

Joan has also become involved with fundraising and charity work in her Fort Worth, Texas, community. "I have recognized over and over that good health is a gift to be treasured," she says. "In the back of my mind, I know that I could get sick again. This thought has helped me live a fuller, richer life."

Elaine

Art has always been integral to Elaine Saltsman's life—she creates art, curates art, teaches art. After being diagnosed with and treated for breast cancer twice, art became integral to her healing, as well. Her experiences with illness—and survival—inspired her to create the chair pictured here, titled "The Healer." She formed the fabric of the chair by weaving gauze with strands of her hair, which she lost during chemotherapy. She constructed the wire frame of the chair by twisting red wire, representing her life, with black wire, representing cancer. The red wire symbolically overtakes the black wire as the chair comes together. "Triumph!" says Elaine. "I'm alive and well."

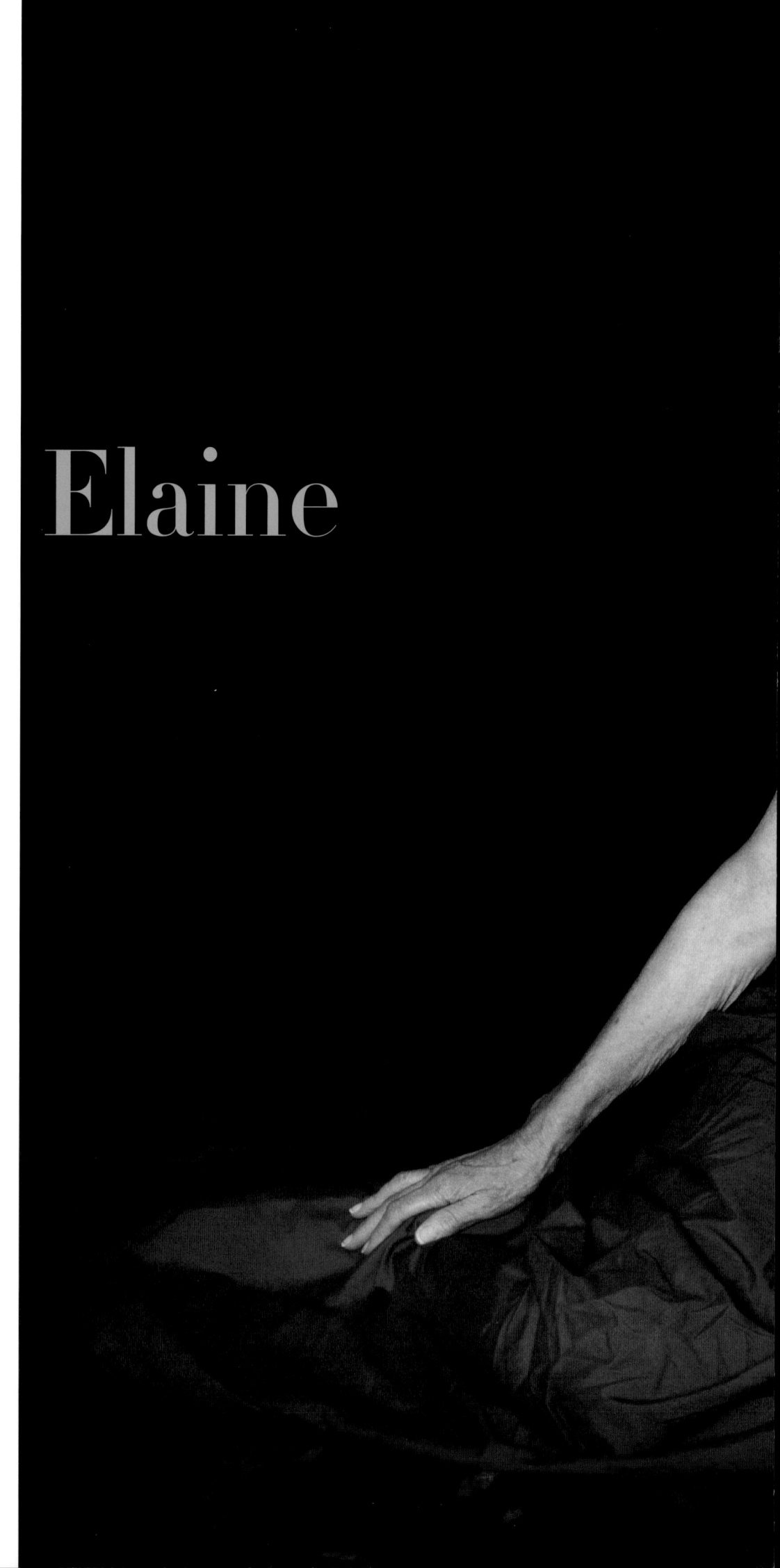

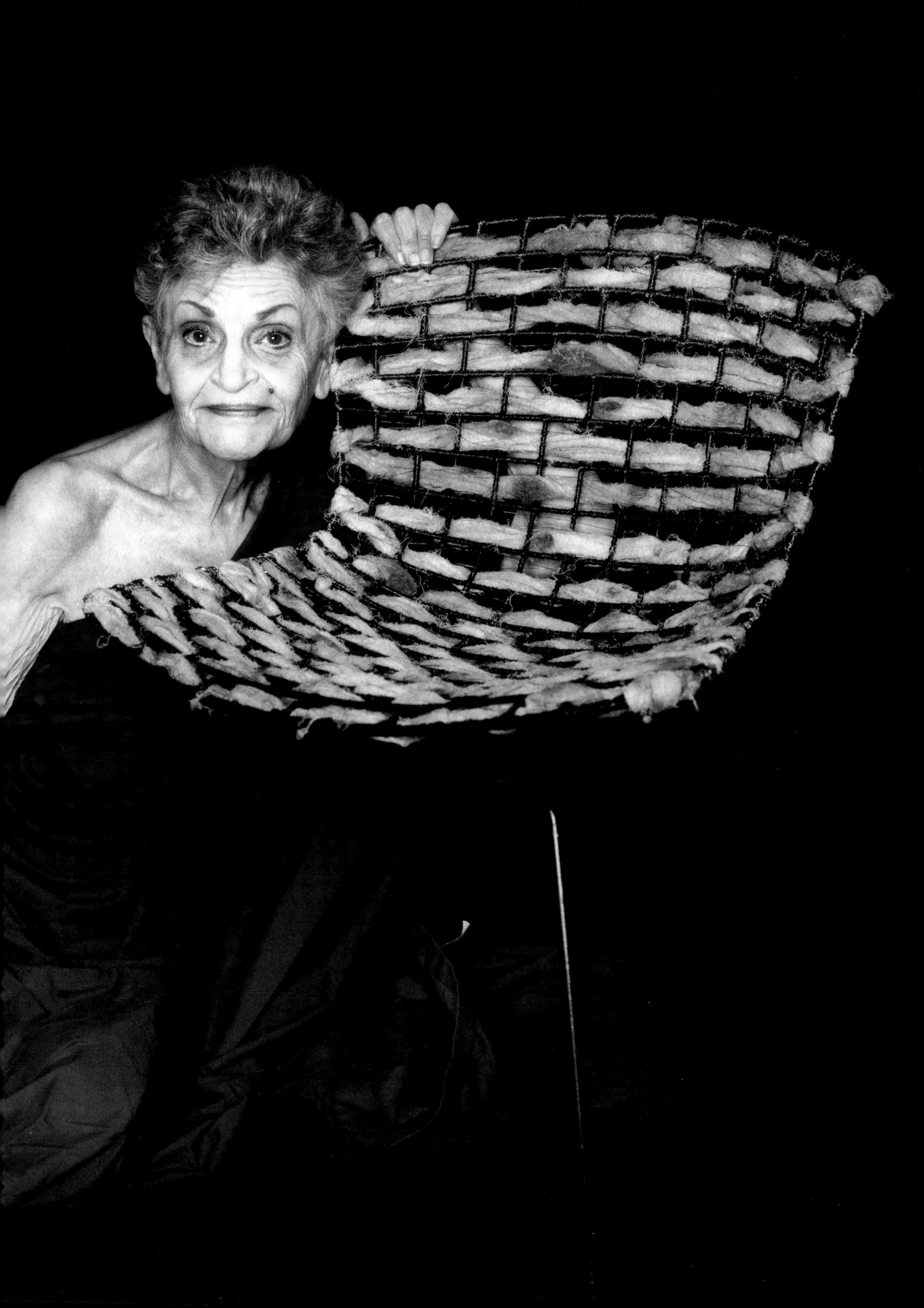

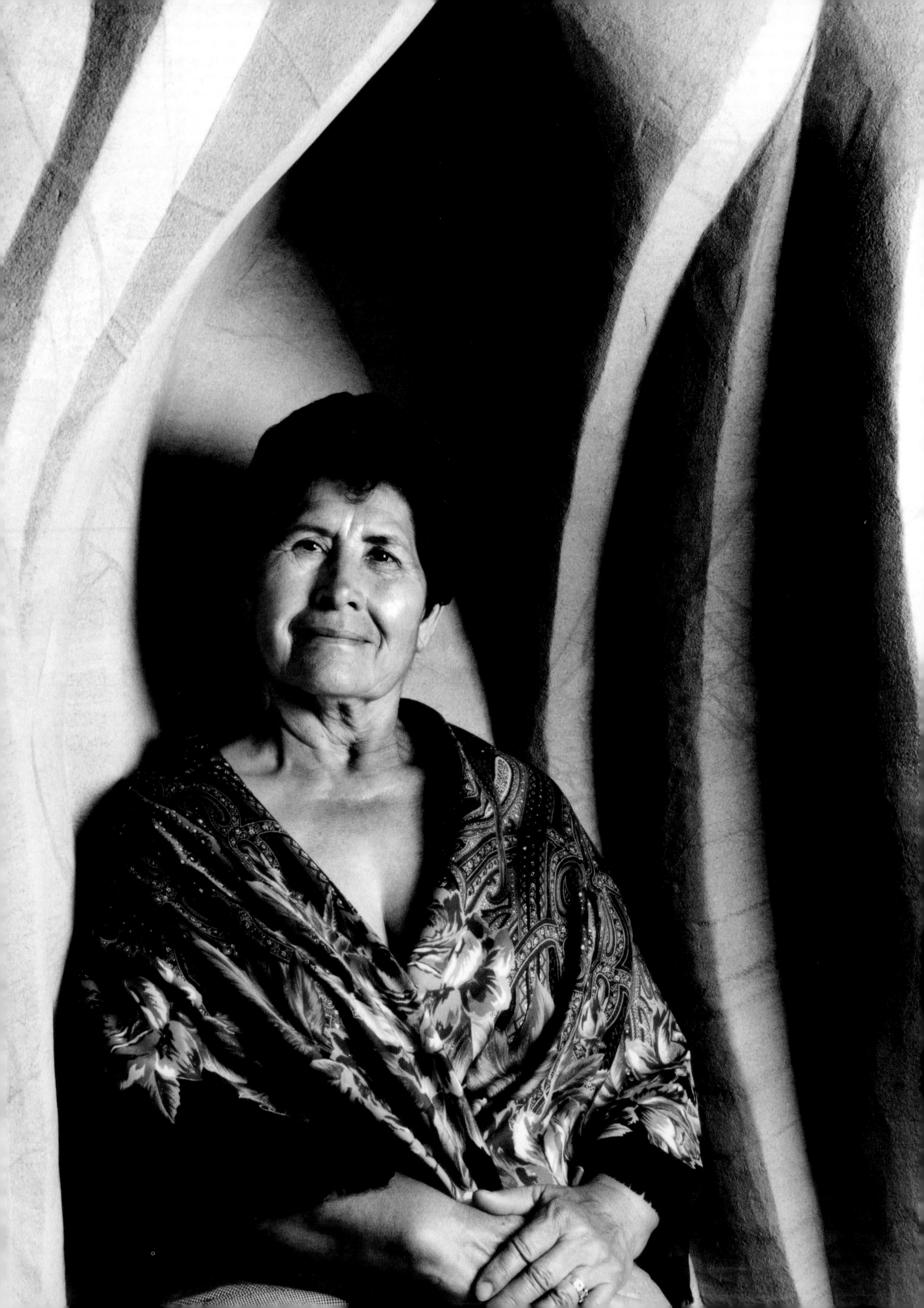

Dottie Montoya is a nurse practitioner in Verlarde, New Mexico. Part of her focus is in helping other Hispanic women in her community deal with breast cancer, offering both education and counseling. She says that Hispanic women tend to be very private about their bodies and what they are going through, but she tries to help them to open up and reach out to those around them.

Dottie

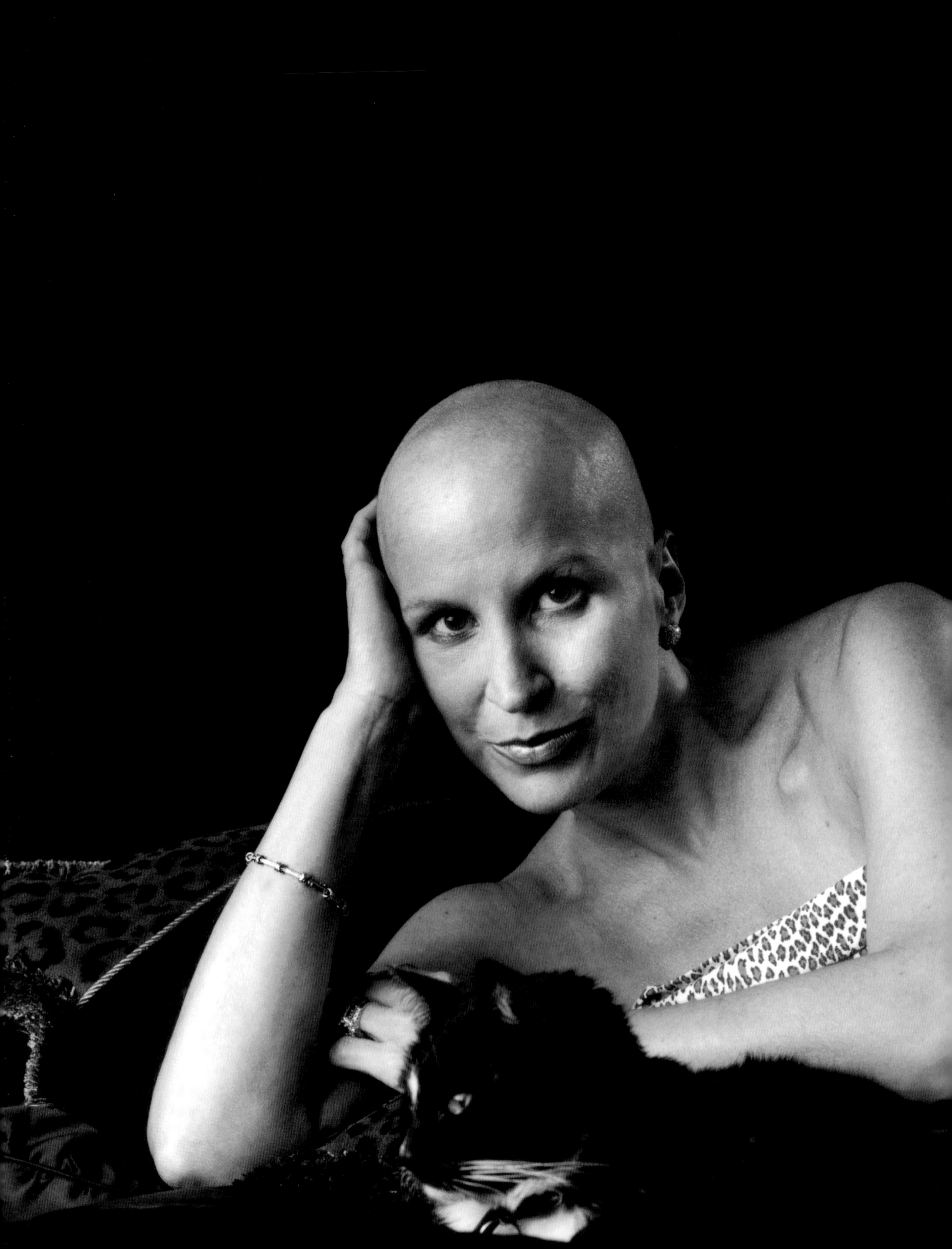

Lisa

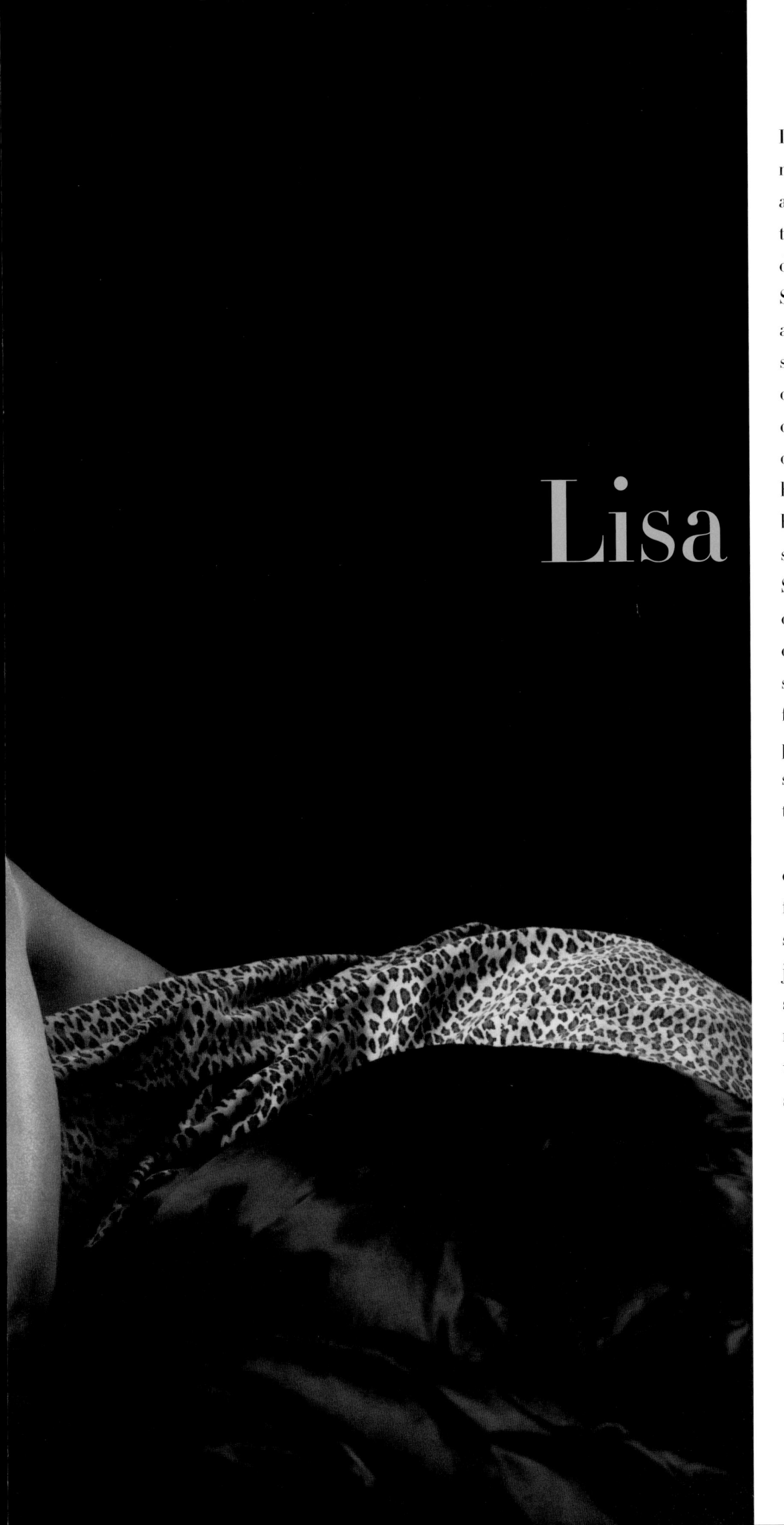

Lisa Conwell was diagnosed with breast cancer at the age of forty-one, two years after the death of her daughter, Samantha, in a tragic car accident. Although she says she has not yet come to terms with her double mastectomy, she continues to strive to see her feminine beauty and her true inner self. As she was cleaning out Samantha's closet, she discovered her daughter's collection of stones. This sparked a new passion for exploring the healing powers of stones, which she then took a step further to designing jewelry.

"In the beginning, cancer was an unwelcome friend," she says. Today, she refers to cancer as just the opposite, and she finds comfort in relating her experience to other women who share her diagnosis.

Gloria

Now that she's a nonagenarian, Gloria Stuart's experience with breast cancer more than twenty years ago is no longer a secret. But at the time, she didn't tell anyone what she was going through—not even her daughter, who learned of her mother's diagnosis for the first time only after her lumpectomy operation. "I didn't want to talk about it," she says simply. "I was a widow. I was living alone. ... As a matter of fact, I had a lover and he never knew it. I didn't tell him until ten years later."

Decades later, the longtime actress (known best for her Oscar-nominated performance as the older version of the character Rose in the movie *Titanic*), artist, and writer still insists it was "no big deal"—and she's been in perfect health ever since she finished her radiation treatment.

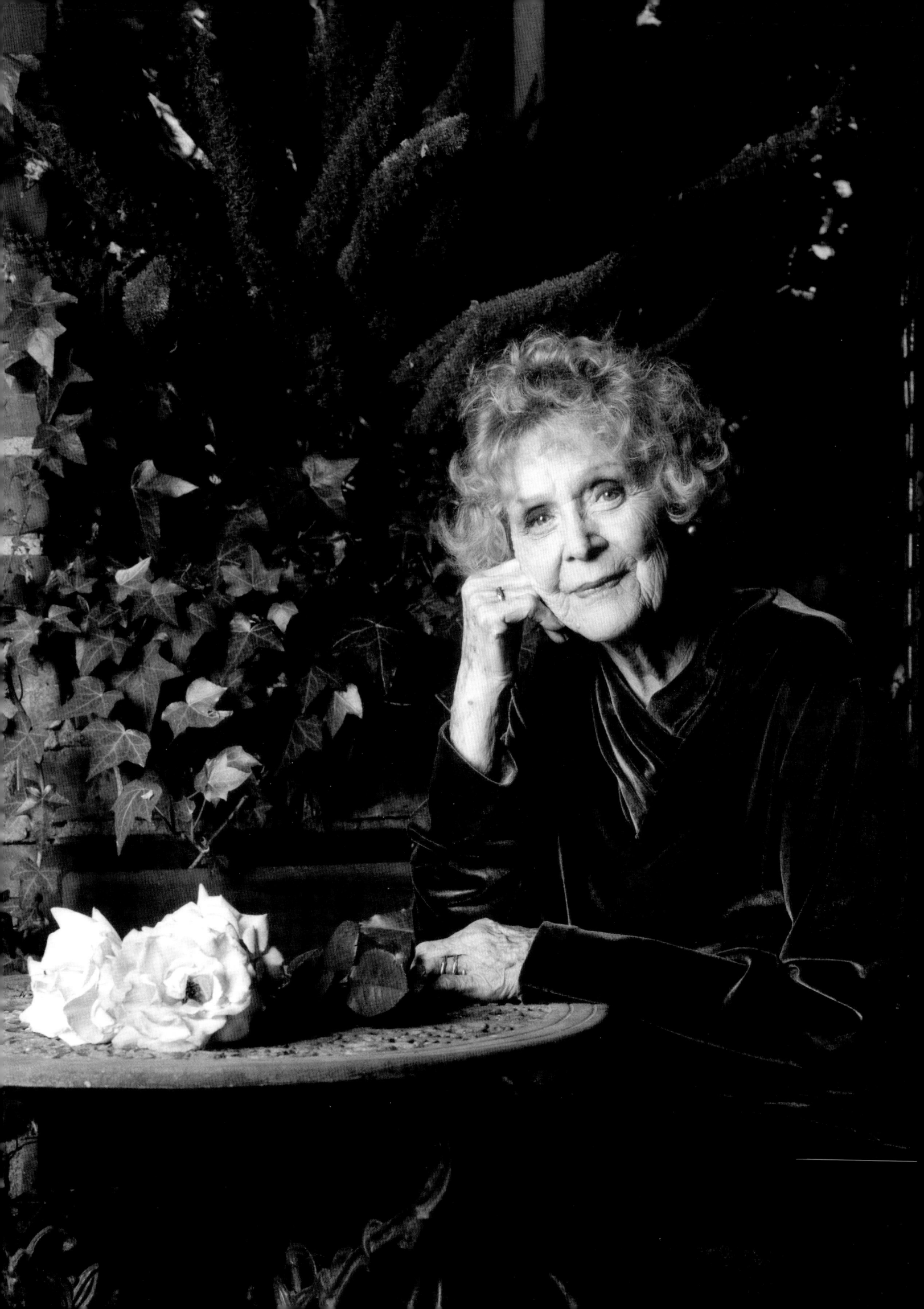

Elyse

In 1995, Elyse Clark was a driven, single thirty-four-year-old working seventy-hour weeks. Chemotherapy cured her of that. "If someone told me, 'I'm sure you never wanted to go through this experience!' I couldn't say I wished this never had happened to me," she admits. "I discovered so many things about myself from having had breast cancer ... an inner strength. I never understood or determined my priorities."

Today, Elyse definitely has her priorities in order. She is president of the Caritas of Austin, Texas, a nonprofit organization that provides food and basic needs to people in times of crisis. And she embraces her single lifestyle. "I am comfortable with who I am. This is part of my identity."

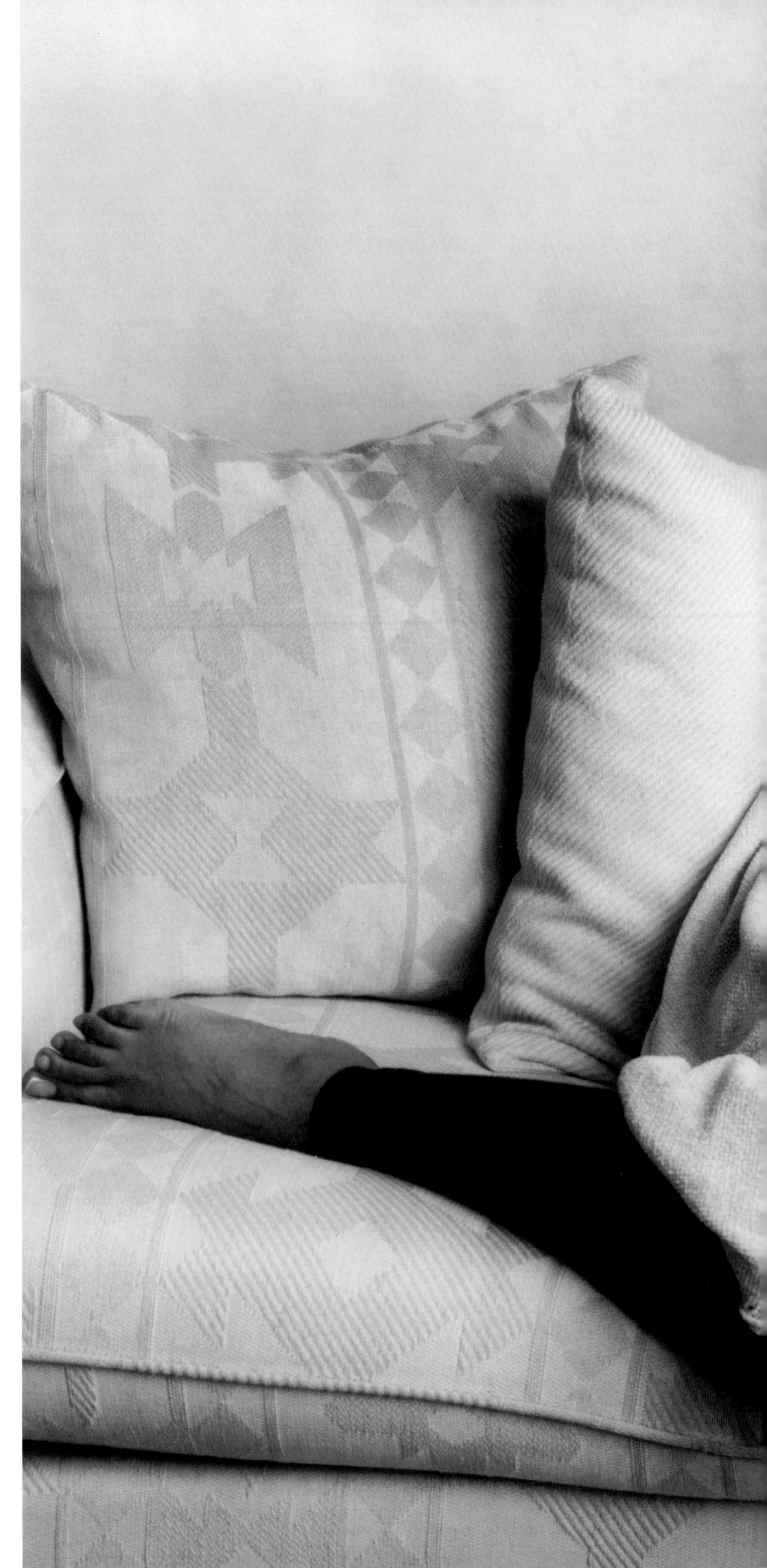

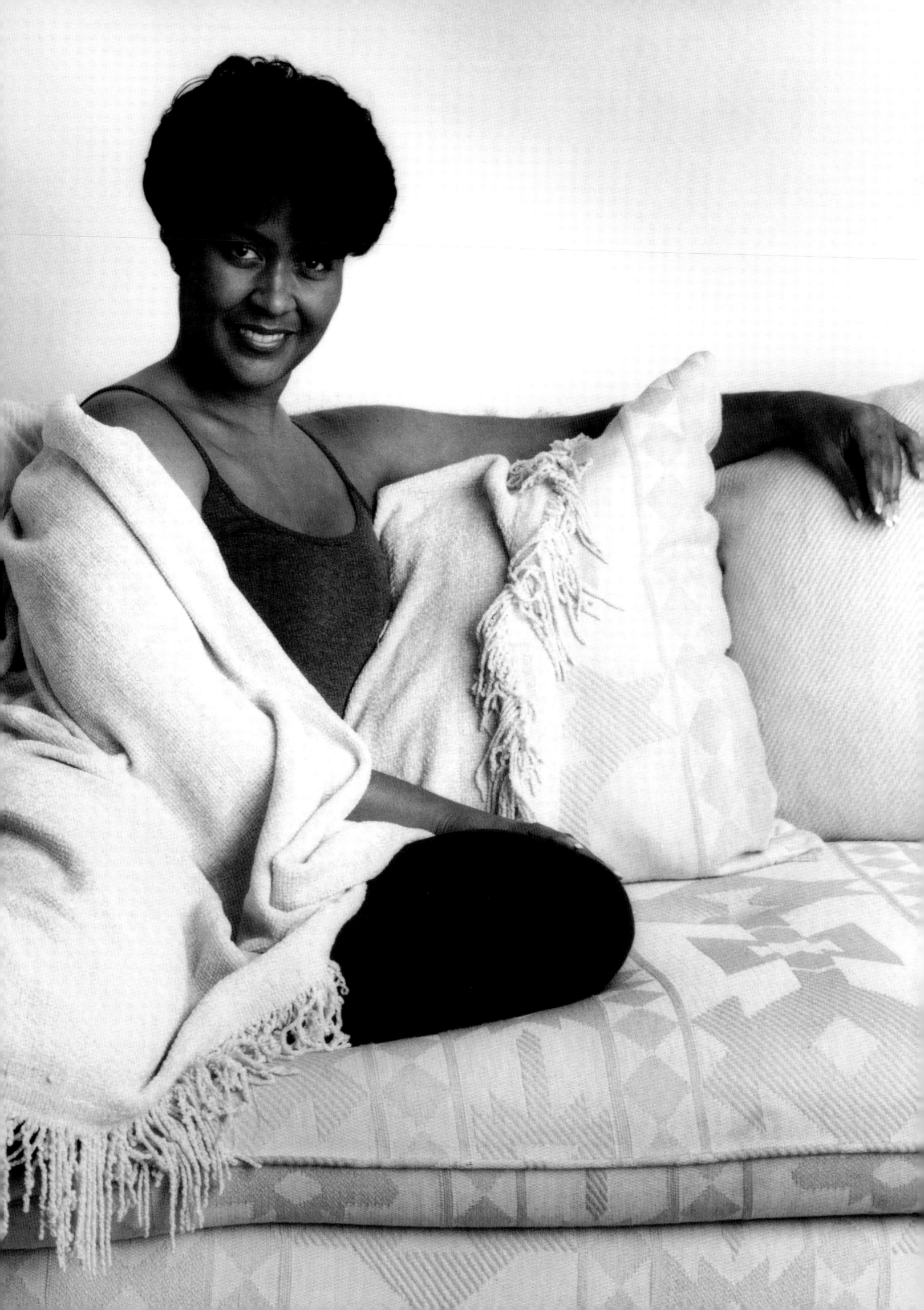

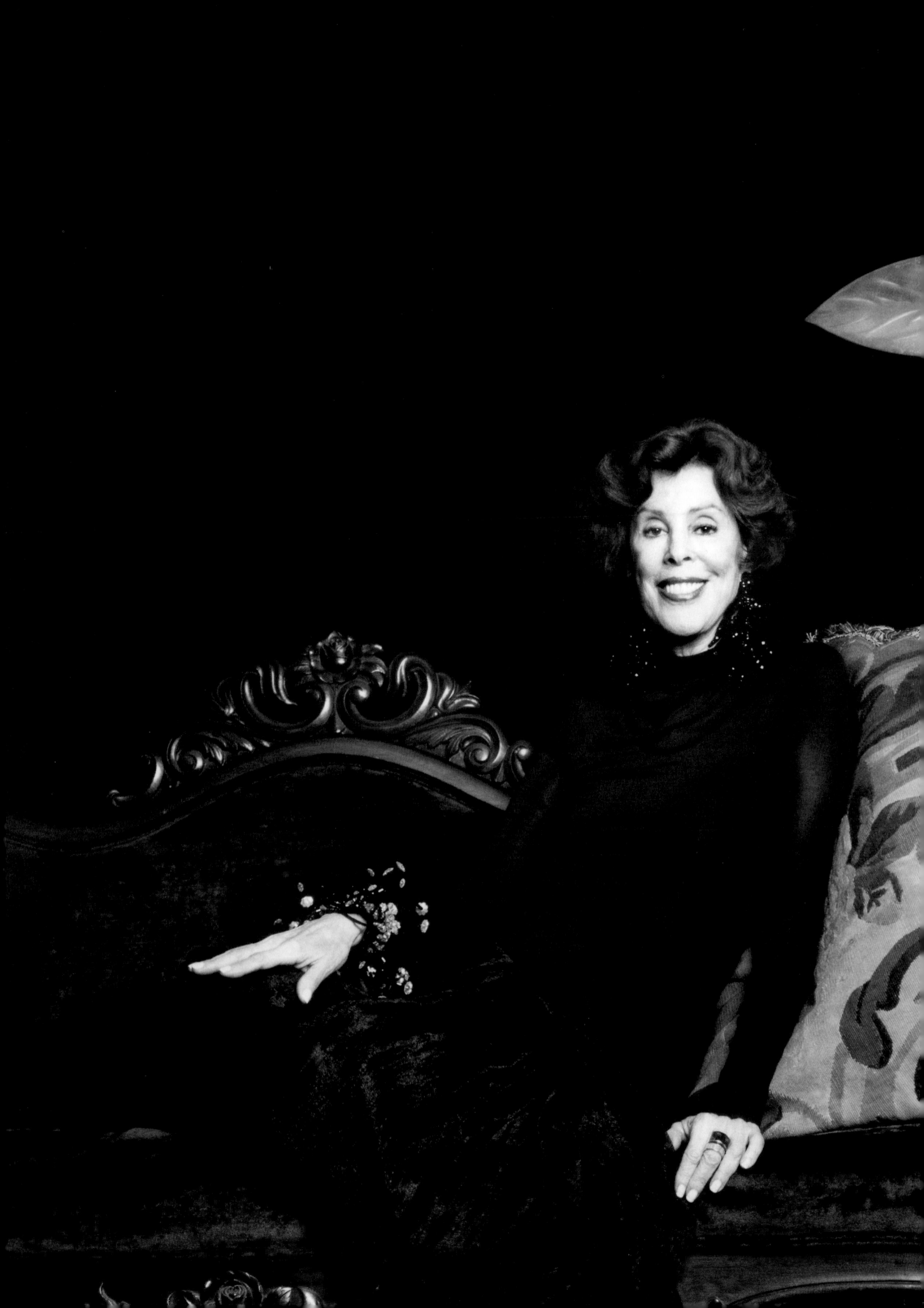

Barbara

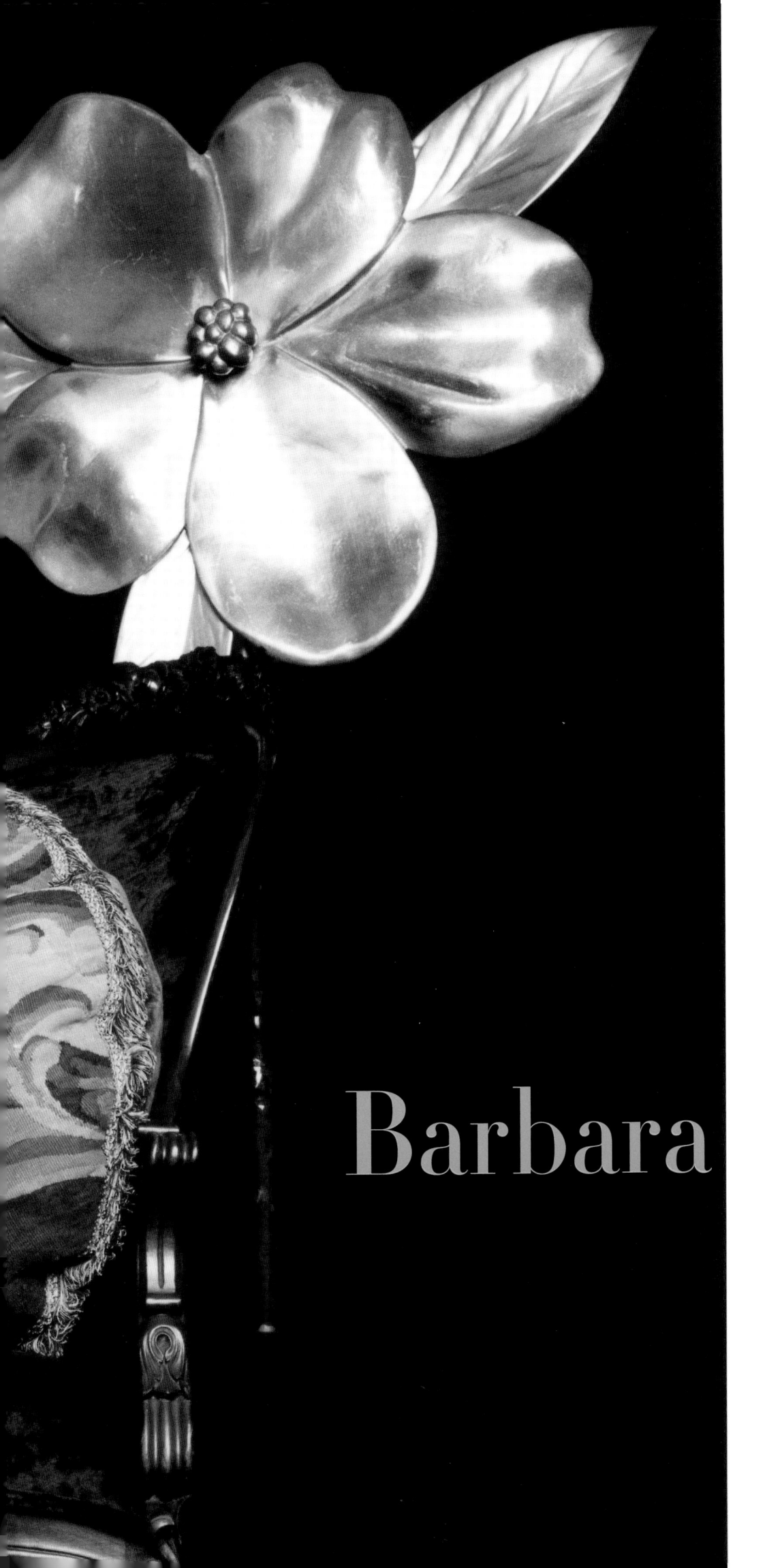

A true New Yorker in the most glamorous sense of the term, Barbara Flood has been modeling since the '70s. Full of great energy and purpose, Barbara says she is always looking for new forms of expression.

She was diagnosed in 2000, and she credits the Big Apple with her recovery. Through it all, she occupied herself with theater, dining, art, dance—all that the city has to offer. "Living well is the best revenge," she says. "Being over the top saved my life. It's that sense of self that wants to survive. That's how to make this okay."

Laura

At thirty-nine, Laura Beattie has been a sergeant with the Dallas Police Department for eighteen years. But her day begins before her duty does, when she wakes to care for her two daughters at 5:30 A.M. She says both her family and her fellow officers—her husband being one of them—offered her complete support through her mastectomy, reconstruction, and treatment.

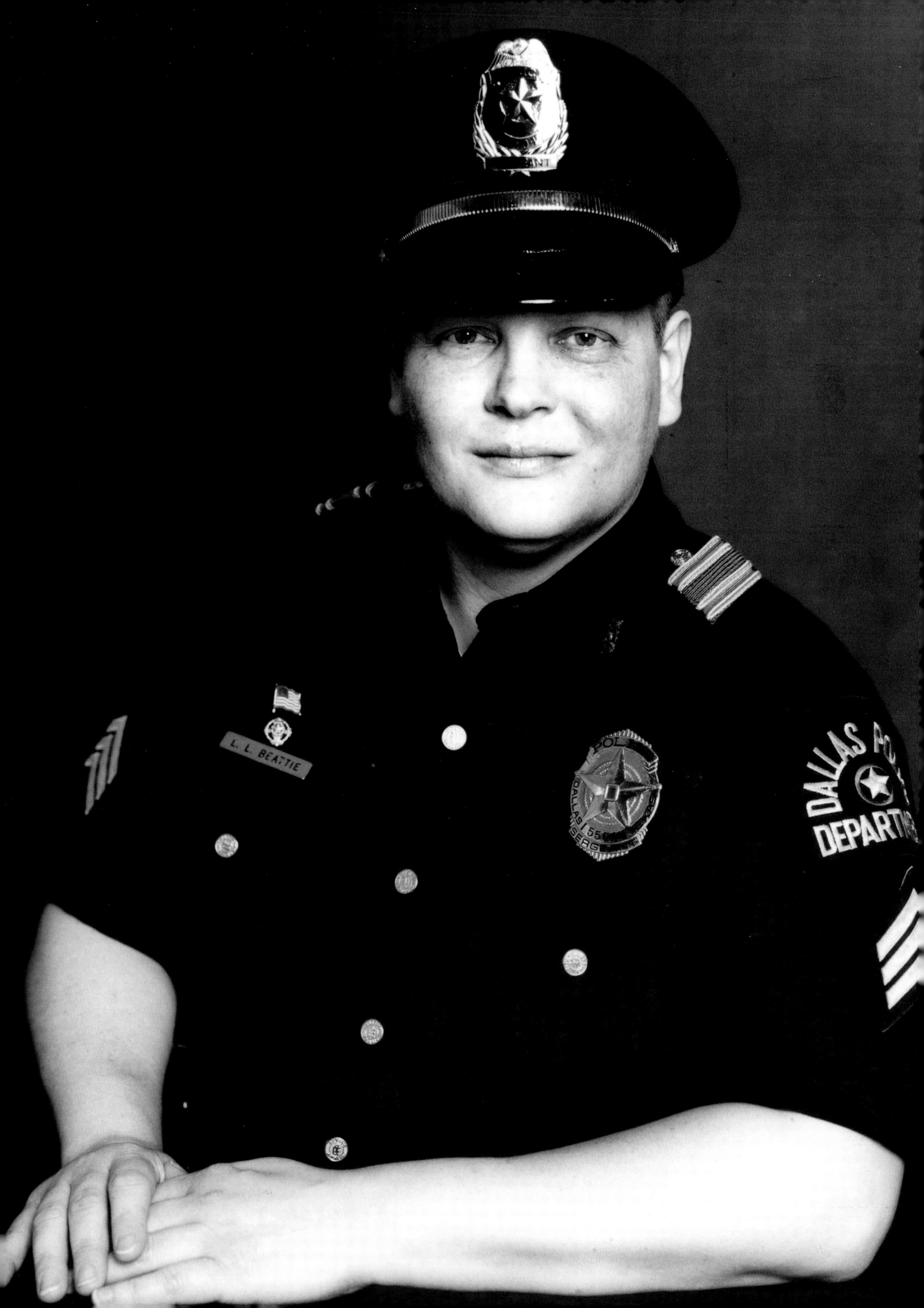

Harley's Angels

Barbara Kelley, Jme Daigle, and Kimen Metzger (pictured from left to right) met each other through the Ladies of Harley group in Houston, Texas, which was formed in 2002 to help put female motorcycle riders into a better light than the "biker chick" stereotype. But these Harley enthusiasts have another purpose: to raise money for breast cancer research. In their first year, they raised $60,000 for their cause by publishing a calendar featuring photos of everyday women who love to ride Harleys.

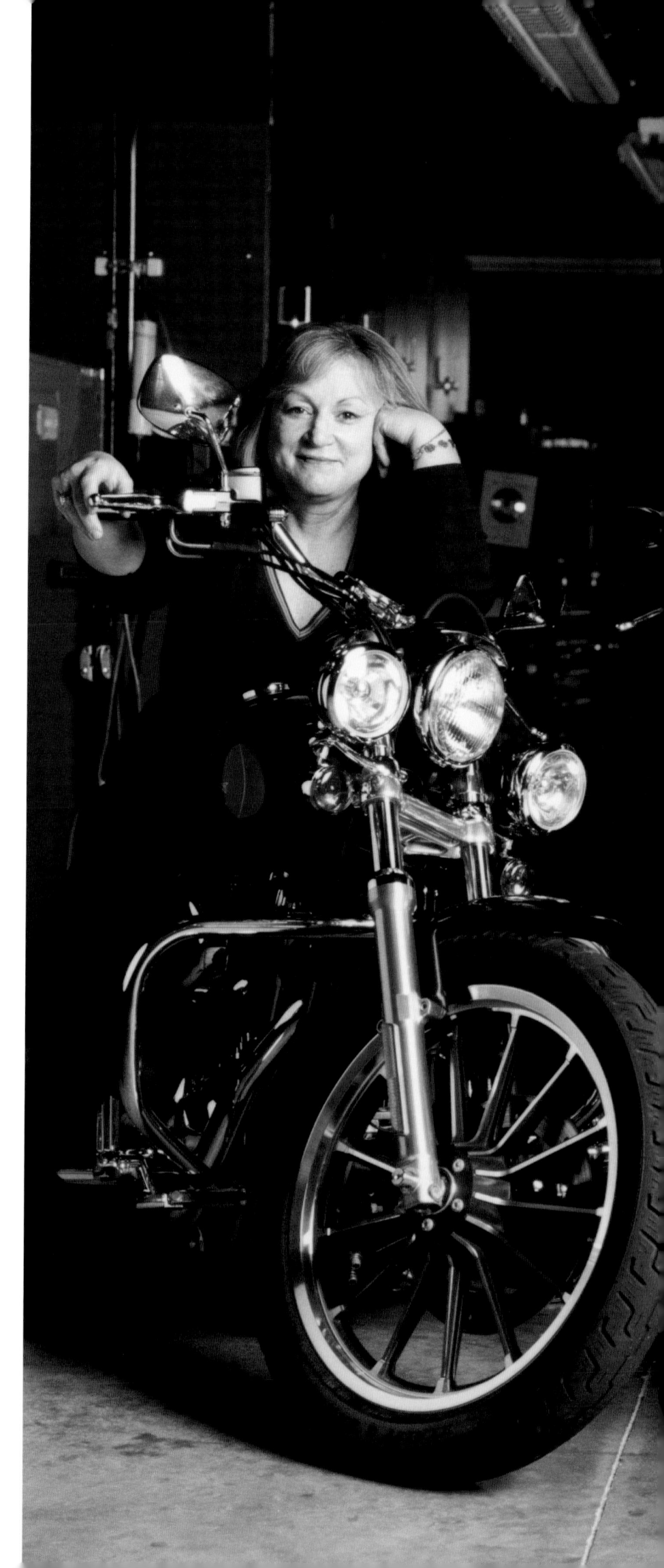

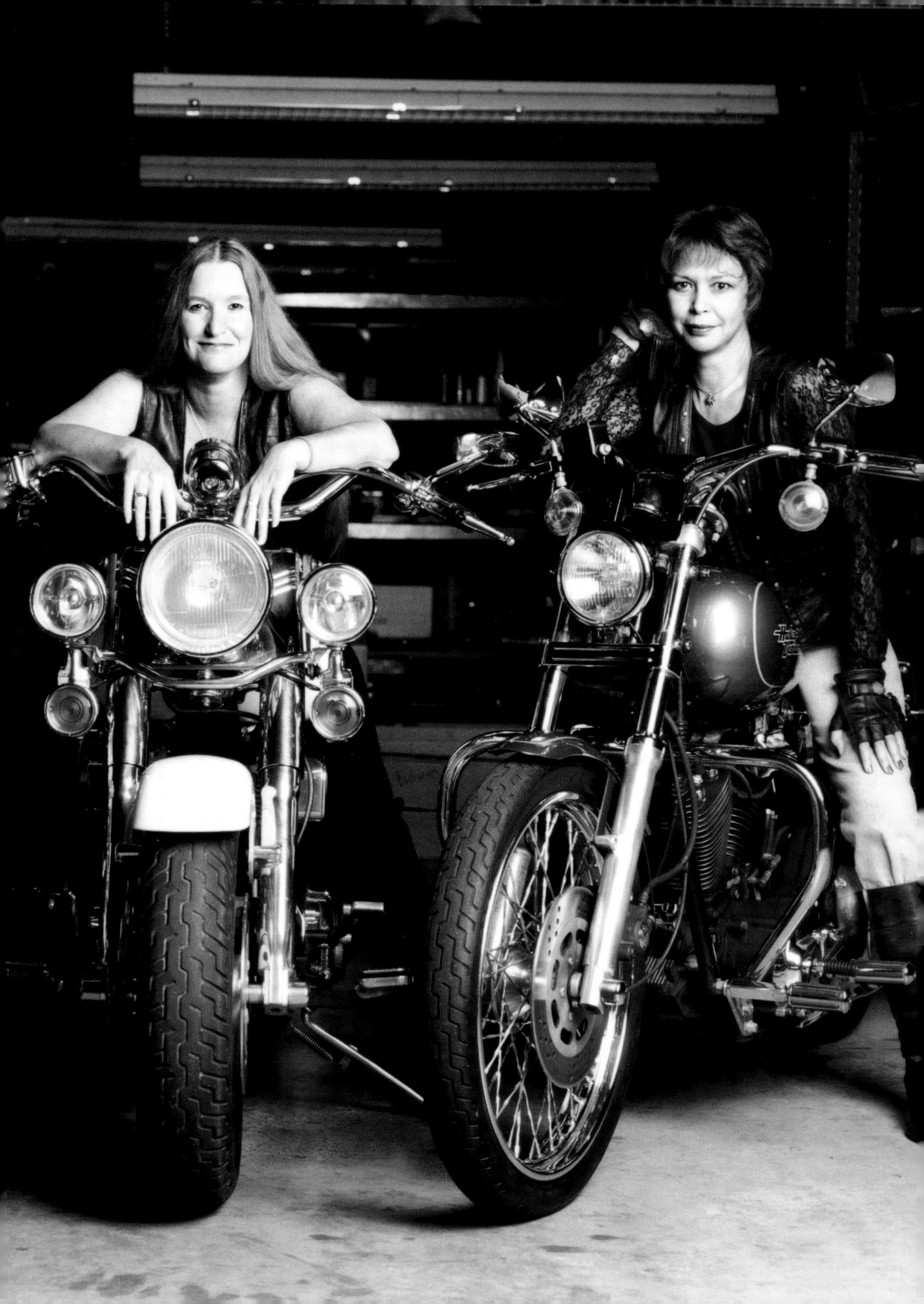

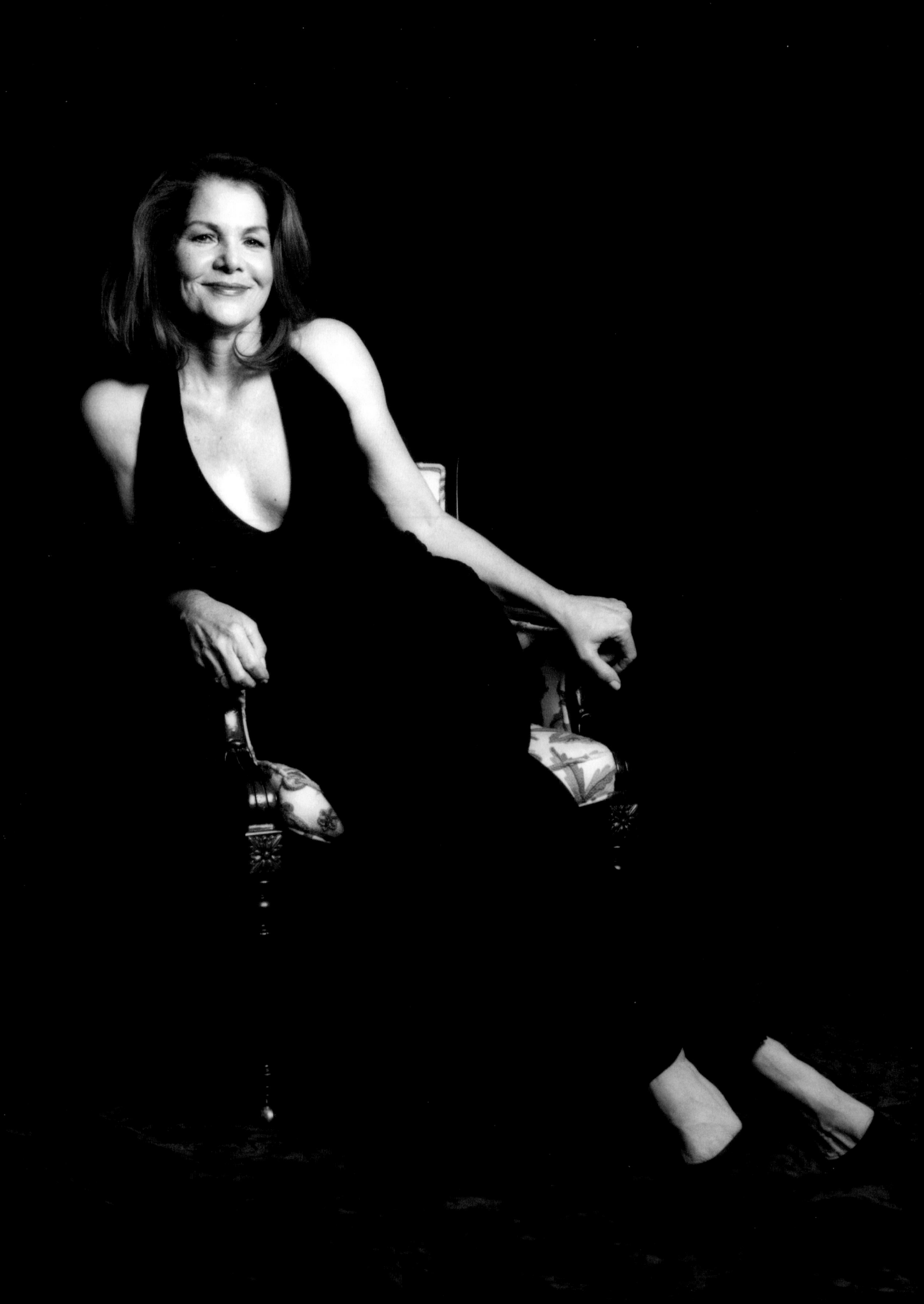

Lois

Lois Chiles became a top model in the '70s, then moved successfully into film—with featured roles in *The Way We Were*, with Robert Redfort and Barbra Streisand; *The Great Gatsby*; and *Moonraker*, as a "Bond girl"—and television—with roles on *Dallas* and other shows. After being diagnosed, she moved from Los Angeles back to Texas, where she had her roots. There, she now teaches film and acting at the University of Houston. Lois has always made herself available as a caregiver to others in need. "I became aware of my own mortality and vulnerability. Now I have learned to receive love."

Susan

Susan Gillette lost her mother to breast cancer in 2002, and after her own diagnosis with the disease, she focused all of her energy on her children. She says her experience with cancer has shifted her priorities, but her family remains at the top of her list. "I've adapted to a simpler lifestyle. There is a sense of freedom," she says. "As my daddy use to say, I don't want to be remembered for the plaques on my walls. I want people to remember that I loved my family more than anything else."

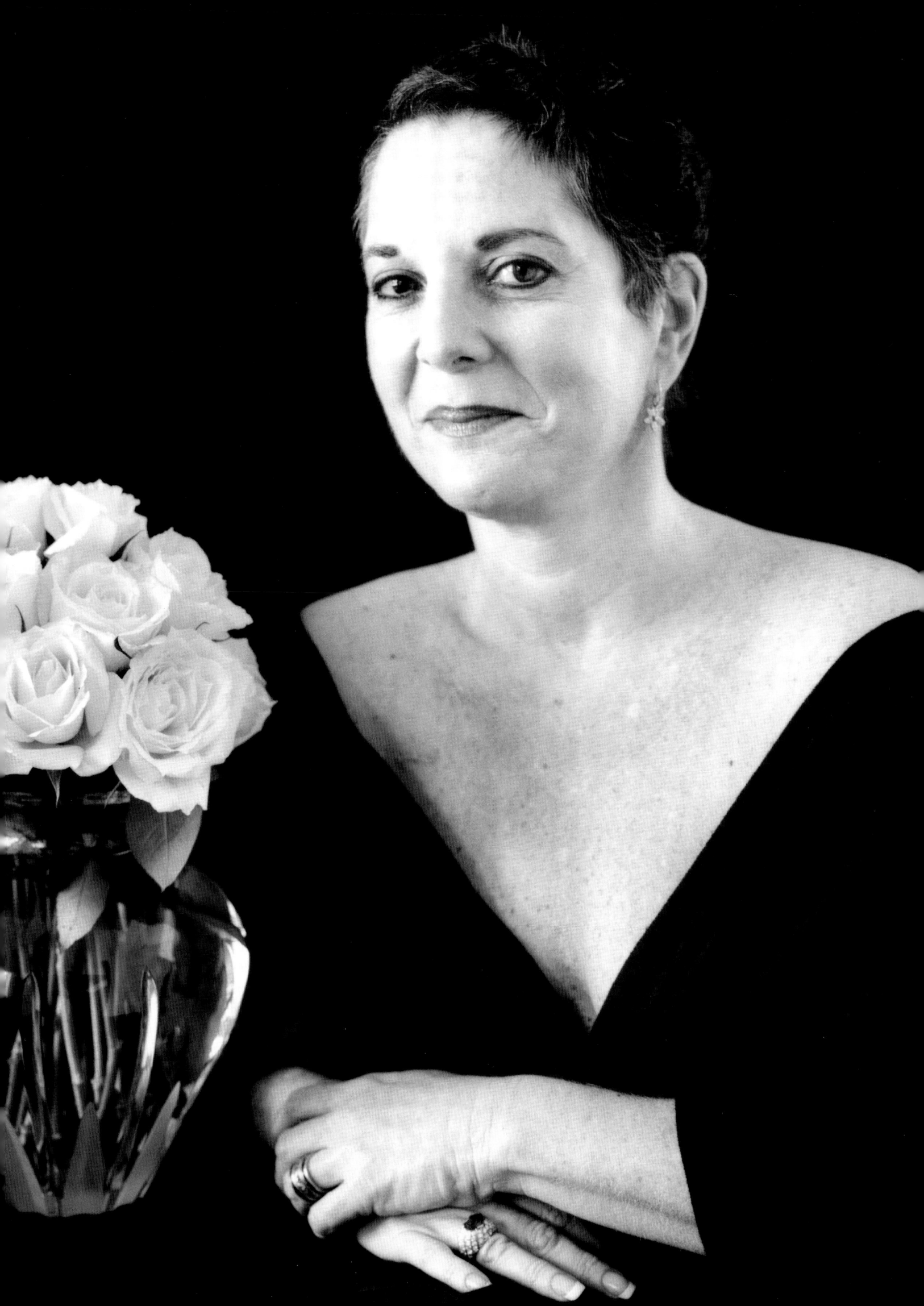

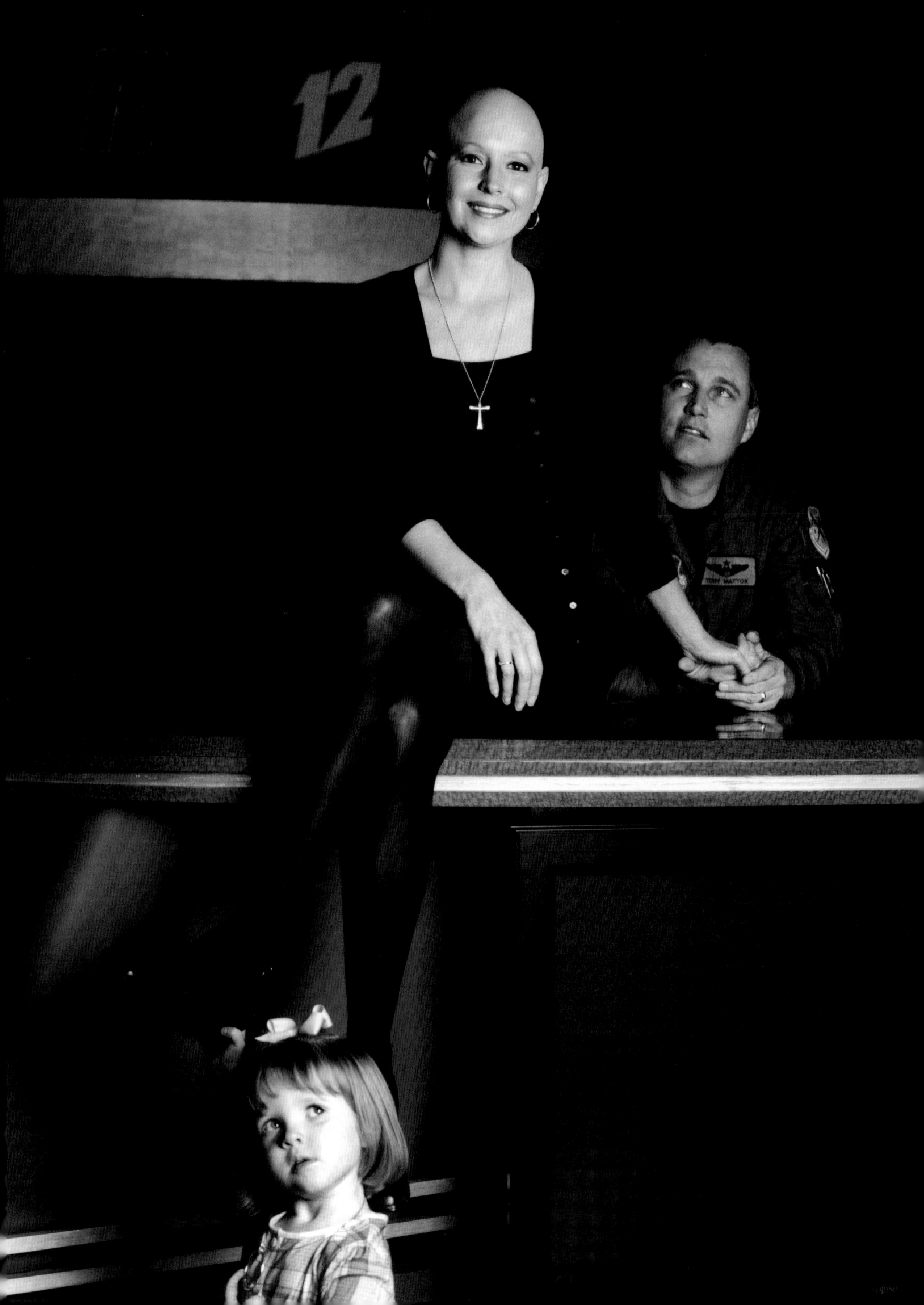

Leslie

A news anchor for KSAT in San Antonio, Texas, Leslie Mouton Mattox discovered a lump during a self-exam when she was thirty-five. Before breast cancer, Leslie often focused on her appearance because of the visibility associated with her career. Losing her hair forced her to look at herself in the mirror one evening and draw a new conclusion: "Big deal! Losing my hair doesn't define who I am," she says. "I learned beauty comes from within. That's where inner growth begins."

Her husband, Tony—pictured here with Leslie and their daughter, Nicole—shaved his head for support during her treatment. To help educate and inspire her viewers, Leslie allowed the station's cameras to follow her through surgery, treatment, chemotherapy, and radiation. She even anchored without her wig during one night's newscast to show other women that "bald can be beautiful."

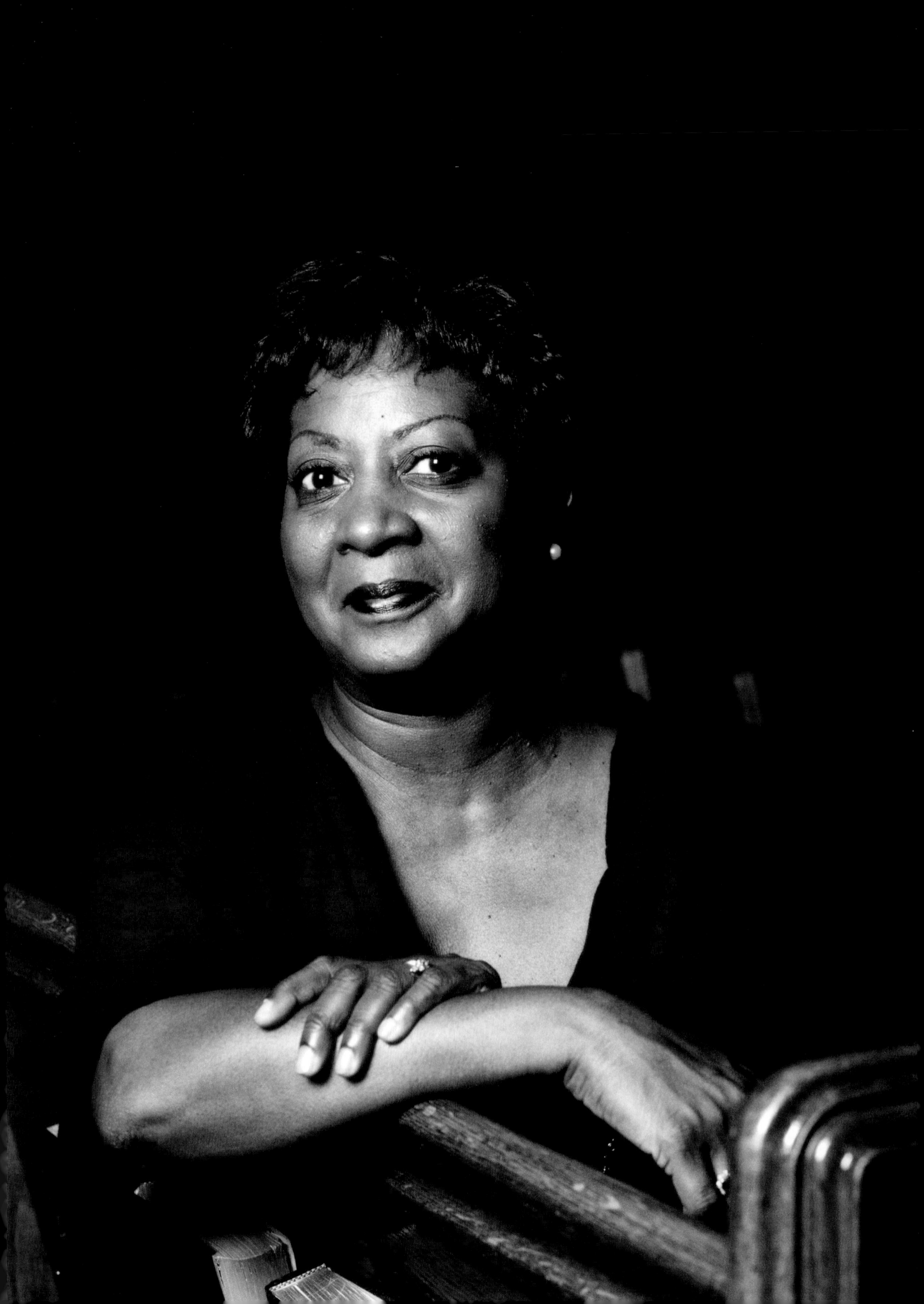

Novella

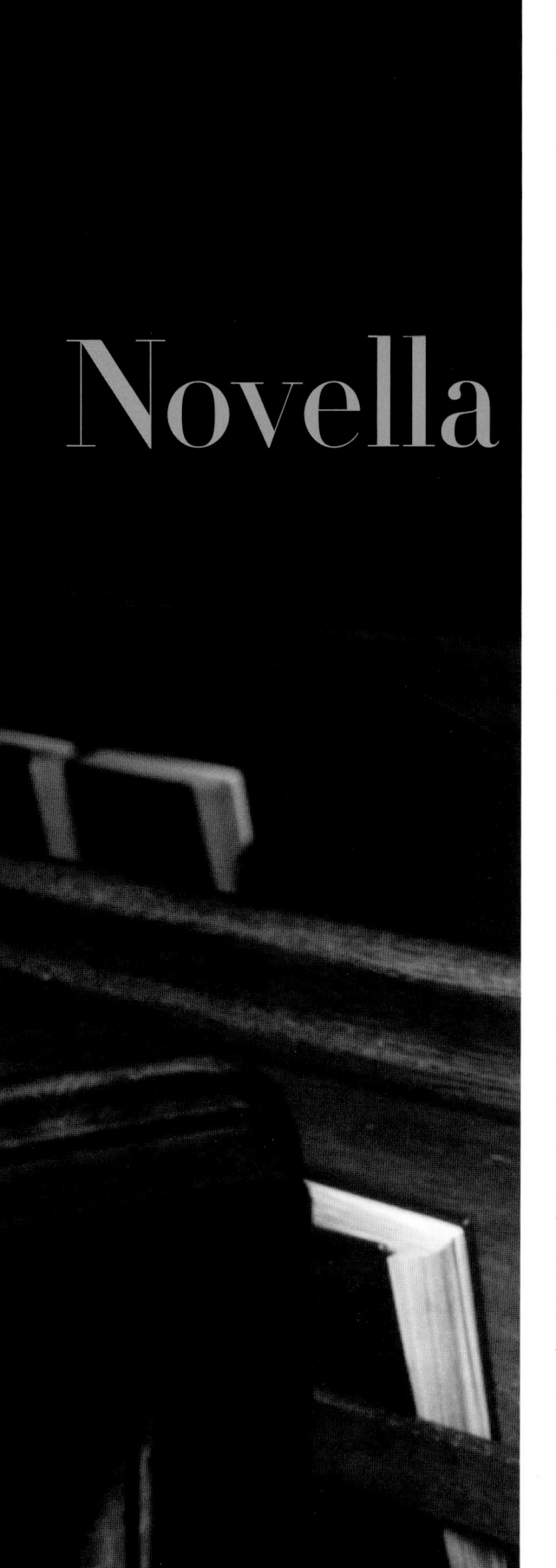

The founder of Women of Faith and Hope, a self-help organization for African-American women in the Philadelphia region, Novella Lyons practices what she preaches, so to speak. She has daily conversations with God, drawing the strength and inspiration to sustain her roles as wife, mother, and grandmother. She is also active in her church, and she devotes as much time as possible to her volunteer work.

Through her own experience with breast cancer, Novella became aware of the lack of knowledge and support among women of color who are diagnosed with the disease. That heightened awareness was her motivation for creating Women of Faith and Hope. Today, she defines herself as living by three words: "Empower, encourage, enlighten."

At seventy-six, Elfriede Gerland hasn't been slowed down by her 1996 breast cancer diagnosis. Instead, she has more than enough energy to go around—and she shares it generously. A native of Northern Germany, she recently was honored for her weekly volunteer efforts at Plattduetsche, a German retirement community near her home in Long Island, New York. Here she is pictured with some of the residents there: from left, Bertha Vidulich, Elfriede, Klara Kluk (deceased), and Erna Gerbel. A grandmother, she also devotes much of her time to babysitting her young grandchildren.

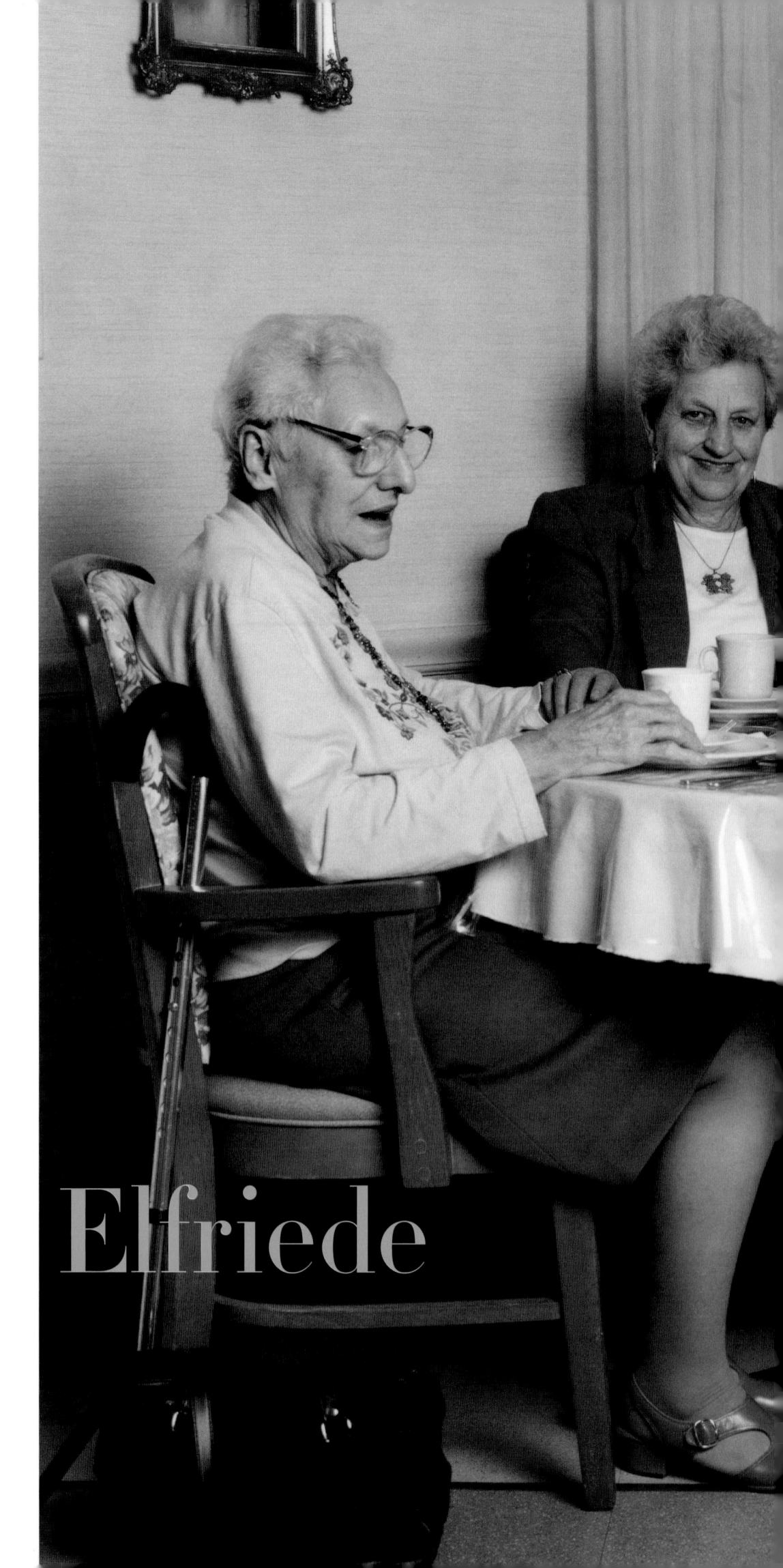

Elfriede

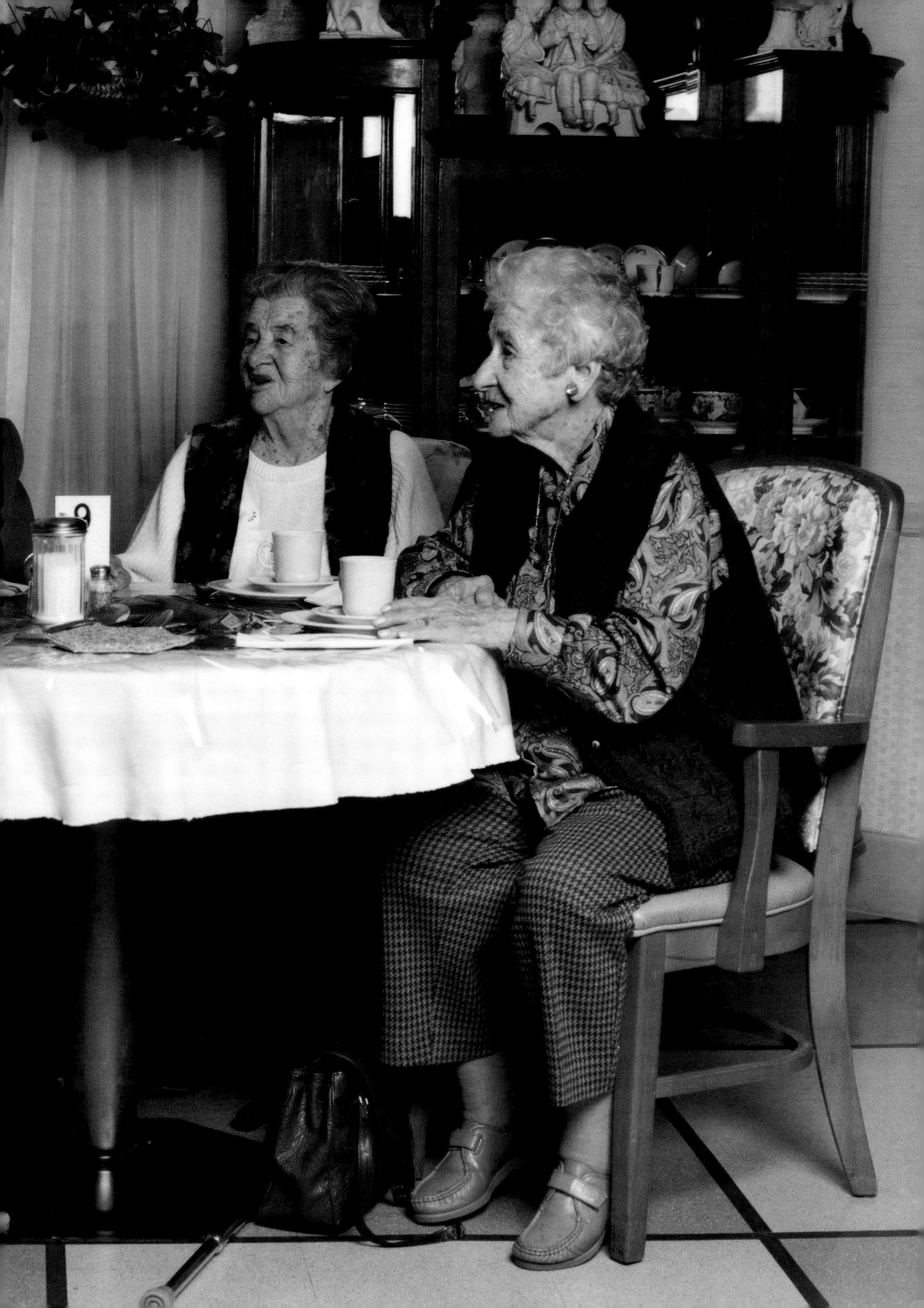

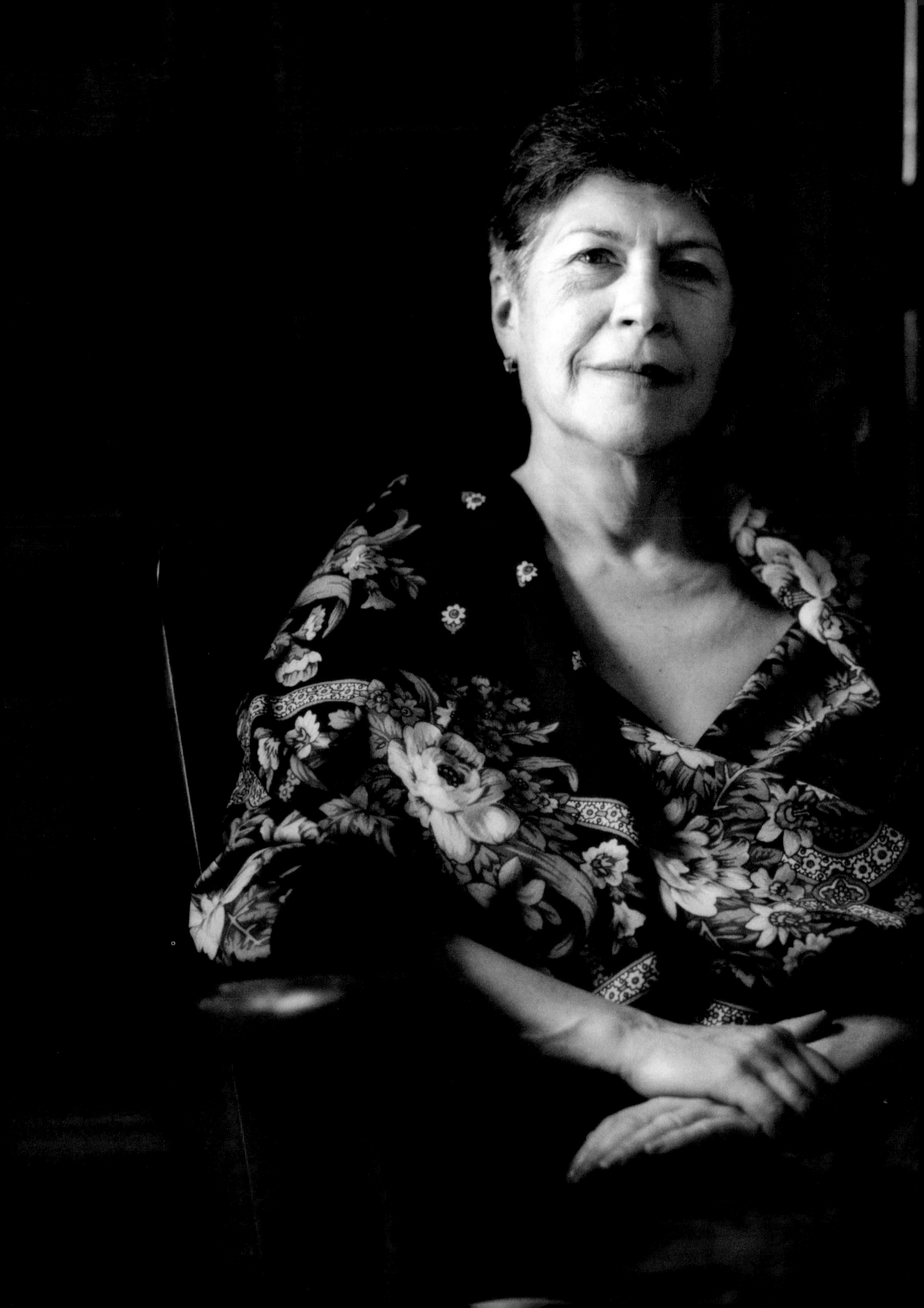

Valentina

A Russian scientist, wife, and mother living in Moscow, Valentina Markusova was devastated when she learned she had breast cancer. But she felt her luck had changed when she was invited to come to the United States to be treated free of charge at the Fox Chase Cancer Center in Philadelphia, Pennsylvania. "It was not easy to go through the treatment," she says, "but every morning I told myself that I am the luckiest cancer patient in all of Russia because I am getting treatment in the U.S.A."

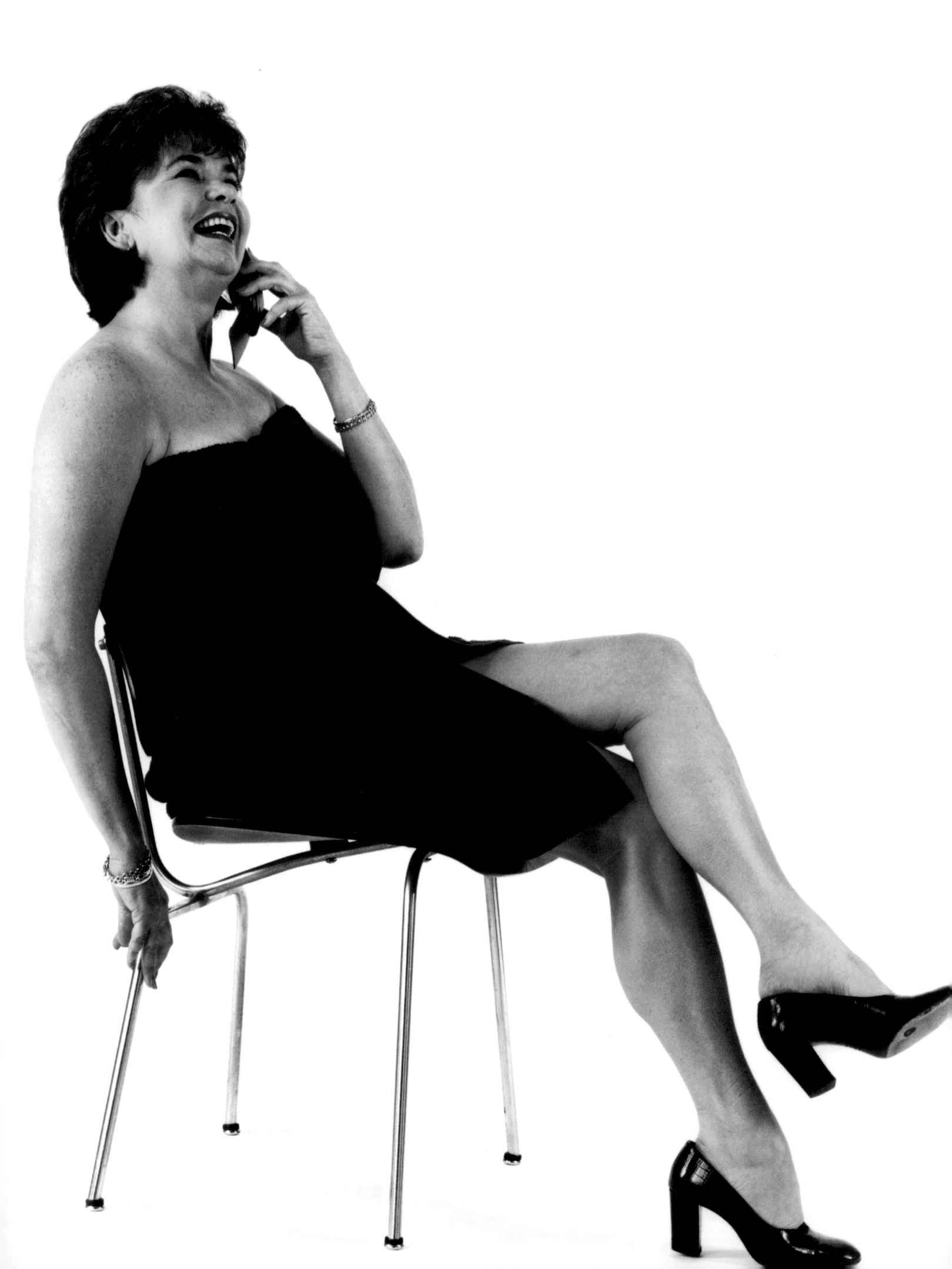

Karen

A role-model problem solver, award-winning business executive, and devoted single mom, **Karen McCulley** also lent her talents to the creation of Common Cares, an organization that provides counseling for cancer patients and their families in the Dallas, Texas, area. Famous among her colleagues for saying "There is no Option B," Karen helped people take control of their lives in the aftermath of their diagnoses, working from her hospital bed even as she was struggling with breast cancer on her own. Her goal was to help others going through experiences like hers to understand cancer, make decisions about their health, and move forward. *Karen died in April 2003 at the age of fifty-four.*

Jill

Jill remembers lying in the hospital room, tubes running in and out of her body, half-covered by a hospital gown. "Being a visual person made it worse," the artist says of her experiences during recovery. She describes the hideous light in her tiny room, the slit of a window with a view of only another wall, and the morphine dreams. For her, the stem cell transplant was a time of absolute rock-bottom helplessness and despair.

Two years into her recovery, she credits the ordeal with renewing her vision. "There were interior shifts in my soul—my choices were revealed," she says. "Before I was sick, self-doubt was as thick as a cloud. Cancer energized me to do what I was supposed to be doing. I feel terribly creative now."

She compares herself to a field being cut down and plowed so that new things can grow. The metaphor seems particularly fitting for the third-generation Texan, whose current focus is a series of watercolor paintings of flowers.

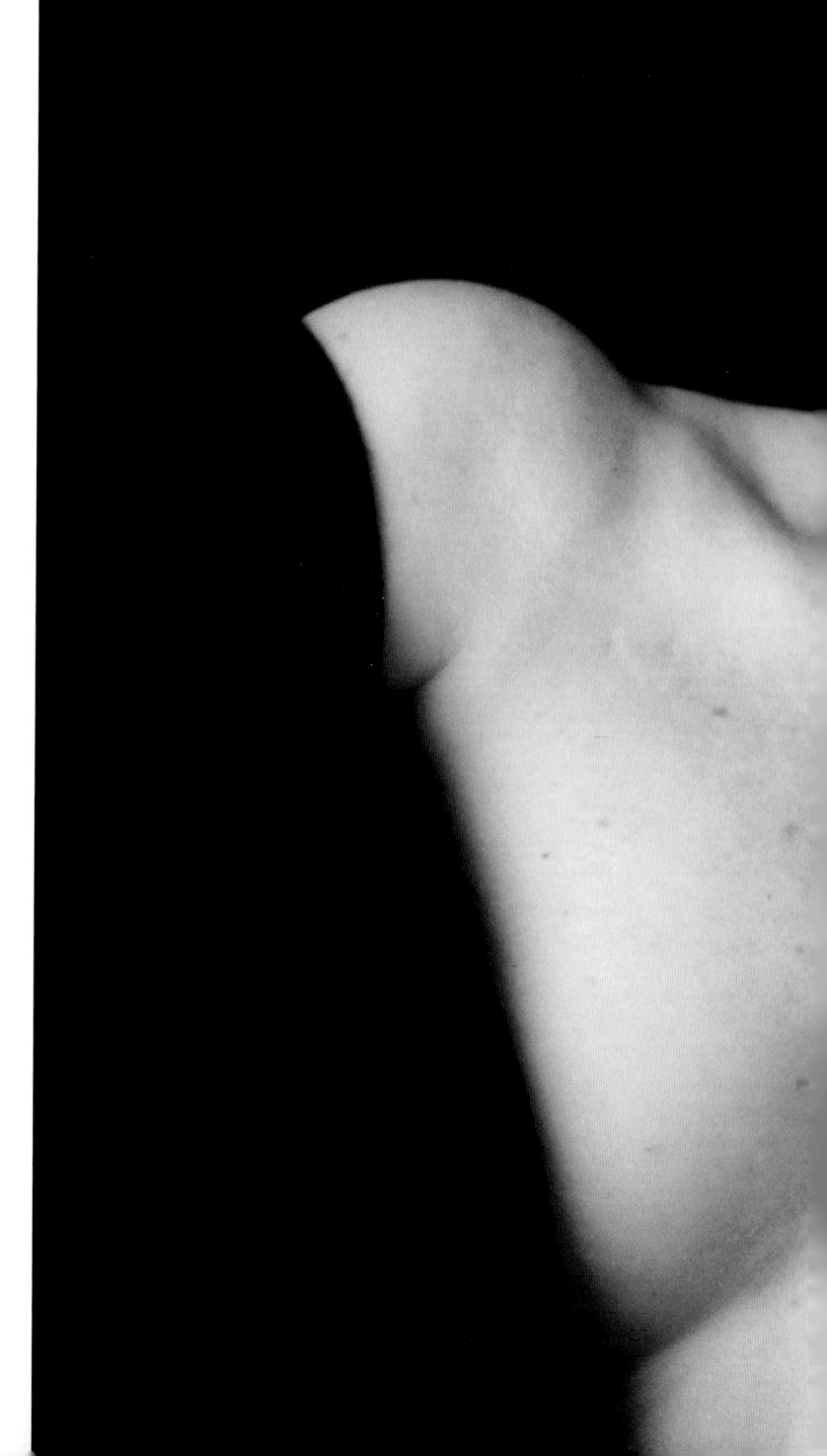

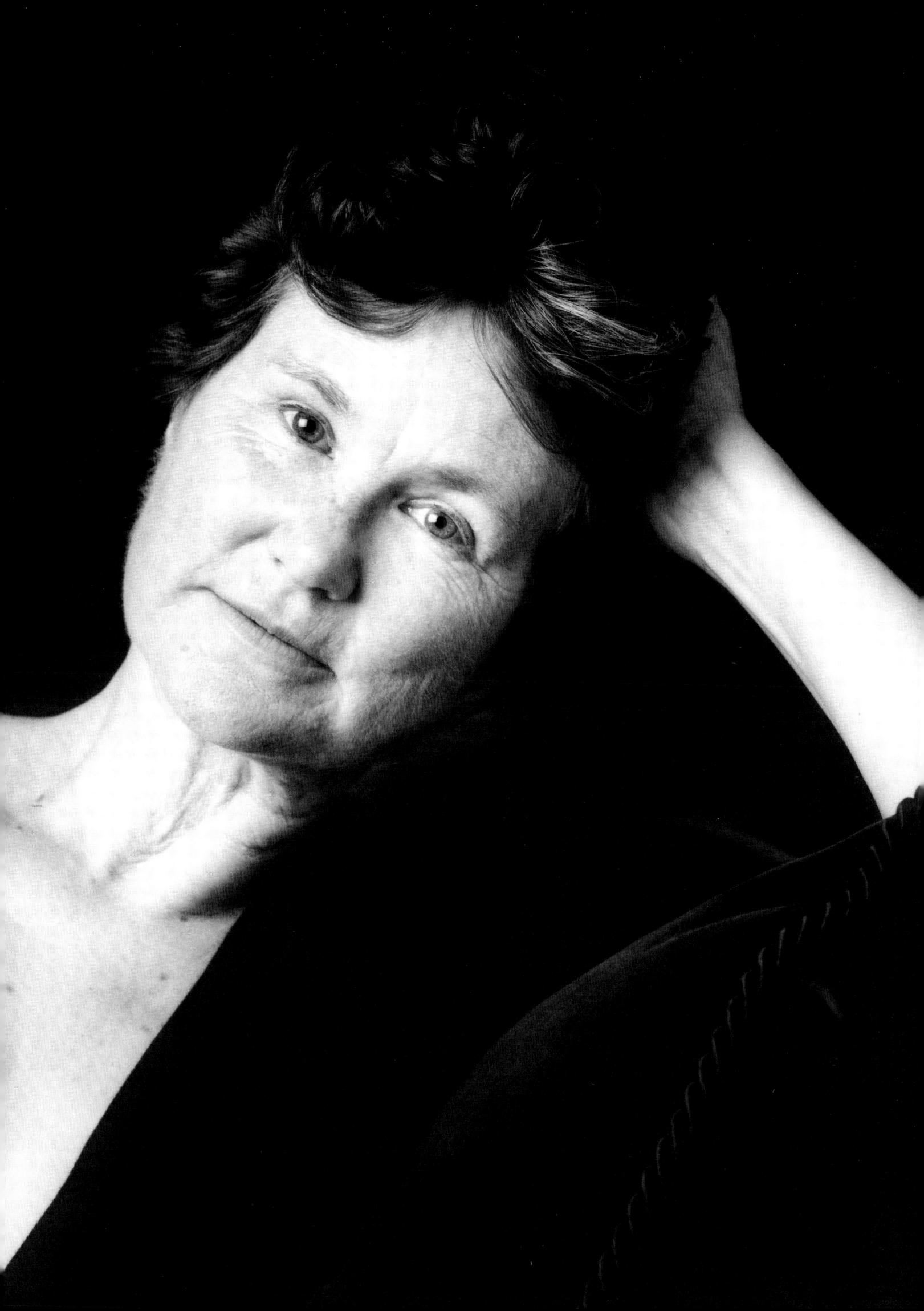

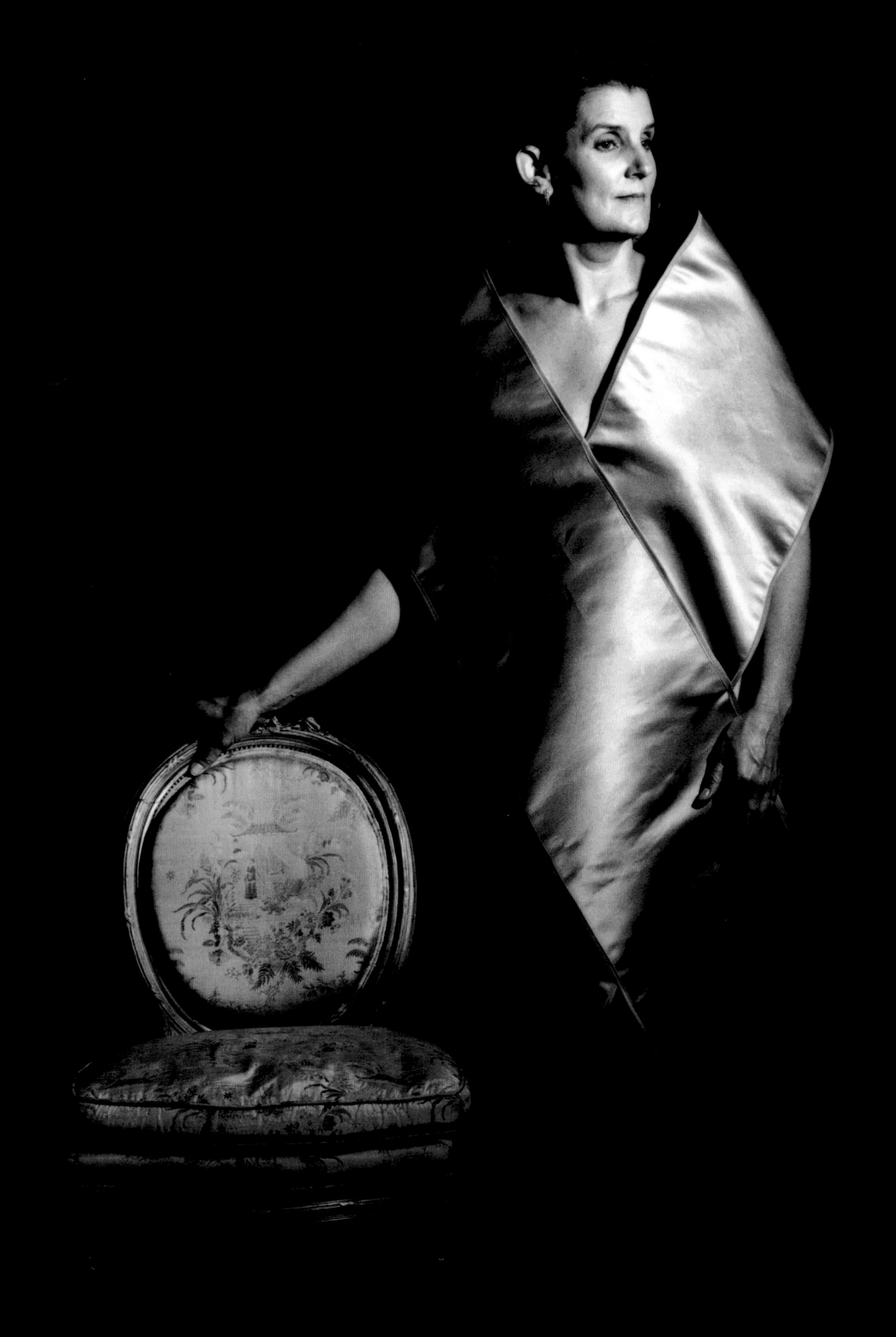

Cynthia

Although twelve years have passed since her battle with cancer ended, Cynthia Hudson still vividly remembers the emotion of her diagnosis. "I was frightened, and felt this was a disease that was not suppose to impact a thirty-four-year-old, healthy mom with a seven-year-old son, my pride and joy," she says.

Cynthia channeled that fear into a new career working for the Susan G. Komen Breast Cancer Foundation, which she says has been a true privilege for the past six years. "I have gone from thinking about my cancer every second of the day to thankfully hardly thinking about it at all. I want to encourage those who are recent survivors and let them know that there is a full life after breast cancer!"

Laurie

Children have always been central in Laurie Jensen's life. She has spent the last twenty-five years as a pediatric nurse, and she now manages the pediatric outpatient services at St. John Hospital and Medical Center in Detroit, Michigan. Laurie's own children—Daniel, Joseph, and Elizabeth—were only eight, four, and two years old when she was diagnosed with stage two ductal breast cancer in 1992 at the age of thirty-six.

Laurie underwent a modified radical mastectomy, reconstruction, and six months of chemotherapy. After her recovery, Laurie went on to finish her master's degree and to receive many awards for her work with various children's organizations in the community.

"Surviving cancer gave me an even greater desire and sense of urgency to have a positive impact in life," she says. "When I was diagnosed with cancer, my greatest fear was that if I died my children would be too young to remember me. Now my children are in their teens, and I hope that they will remember their mother as someone who was committed to helping others."

Here Laurie is pictured with three children for whom she helped care when they were in St. John's neonatal intensive care unit after being born prematurely: Heather Cleland (Christmas tree), Melissa Jones (princess), and Carley Marie Glugla (fairy).

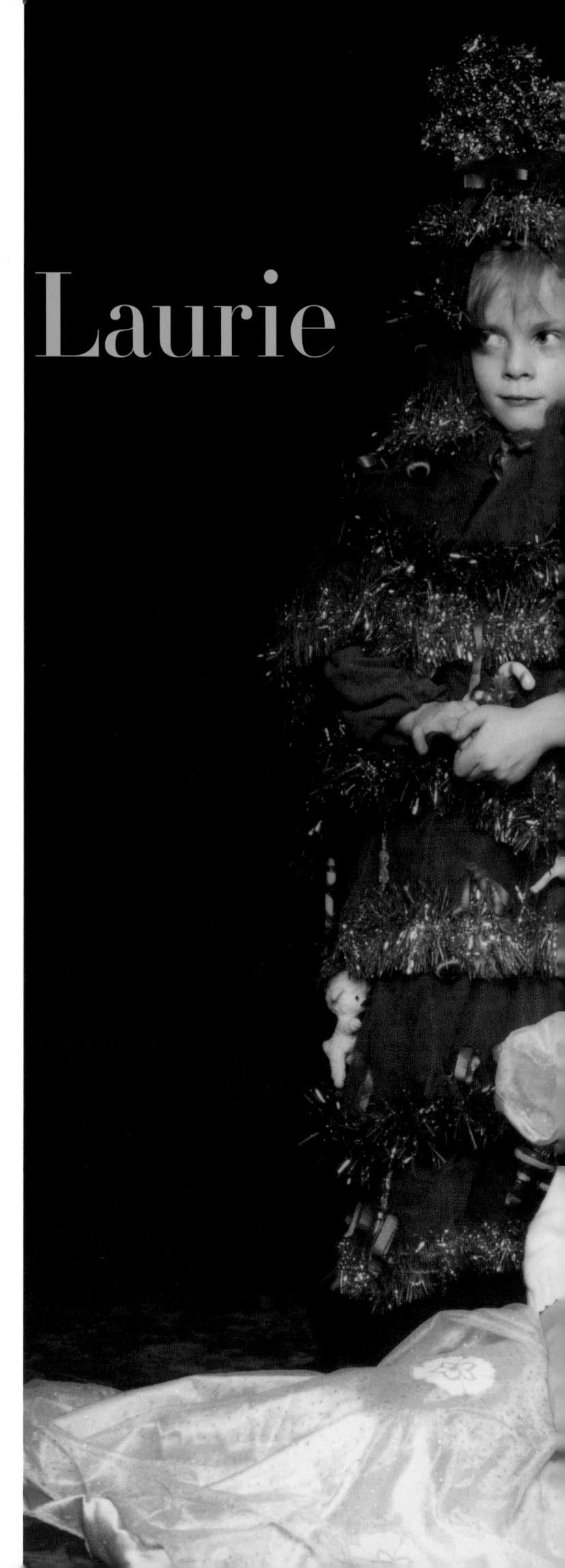

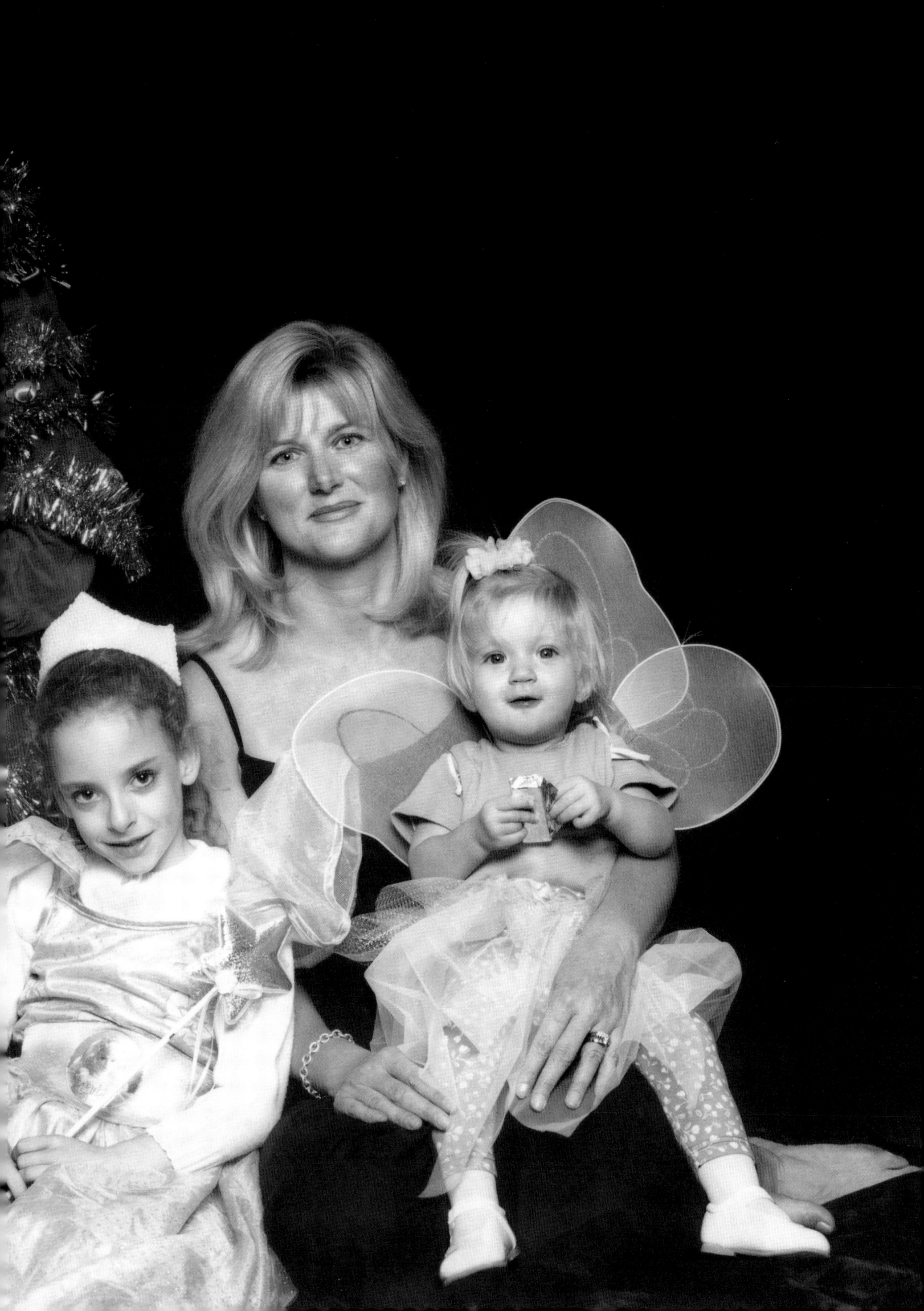

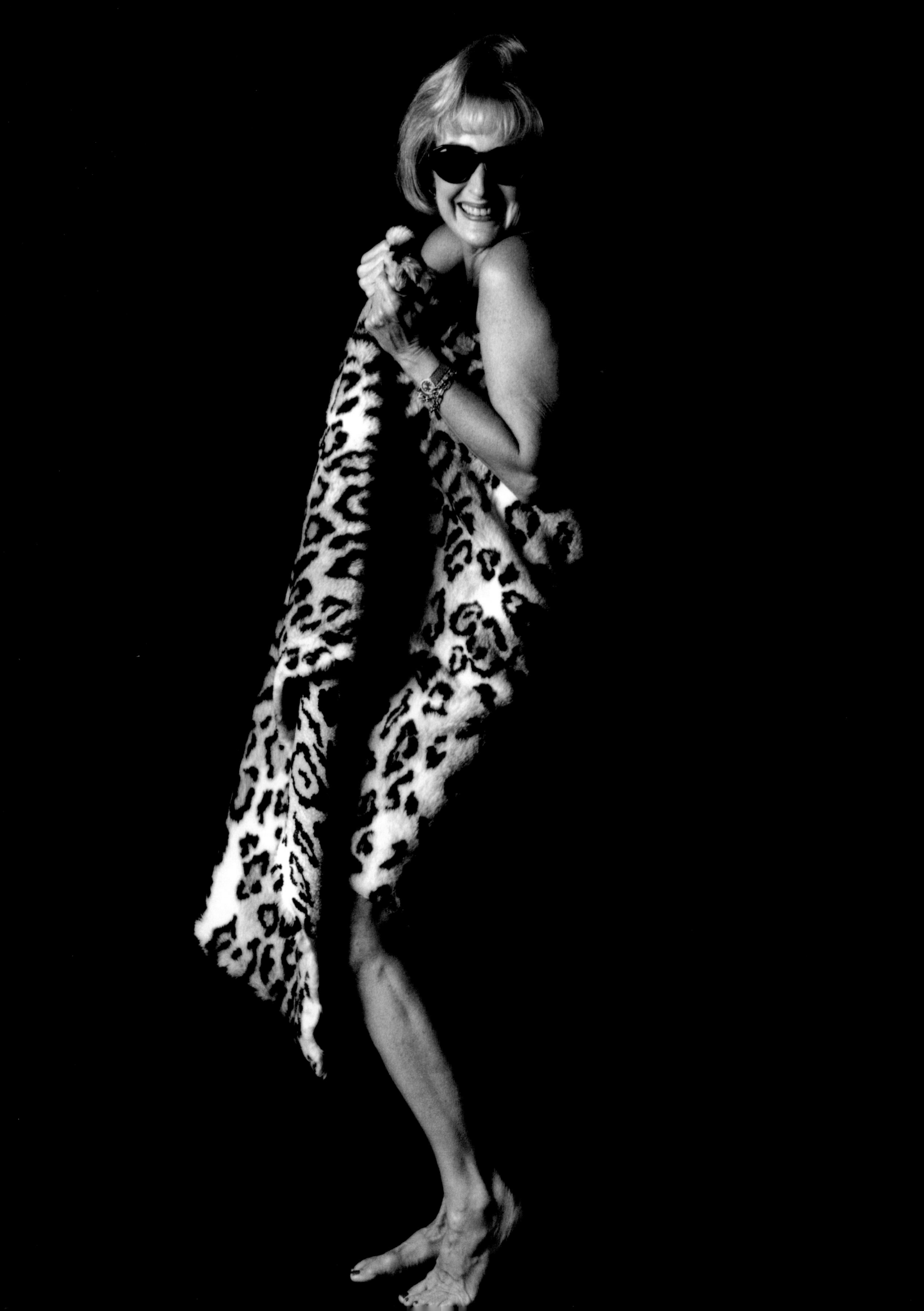

Karen

Breast cancer changed the way Karen Faulkner Key perceived her body; her reconstruction helped bring out her feminine side and her sexuality. As a single woman during that period, Karen says the illness added a difficult dimension to dating. But at age forty-nine, she met and married the man of her dreams. The couple shares a common bond: Each of them experienced—and survived—a life-threatening health problem. "I would never have met the right man if it weren't for breast cancer," she says.

Jana

A breast cancer survivor for seven years now, Jana Johnson looks back on her cancer experience as a whirlwind of racing thoughts and emotions. Her experience culminated at the sixty-mile Avon Walk in Chicago two years ago—she says standing with forty thousand people at the closing ceremony on a Lake Michigan beach gave her the feeling of belonging to a sisterhood.

Today, she works in an intimate apparel shop near her home in Highland Park, Illinois. At least 10 percent of her customers are dealing with breast cancer, and Jana and her co-workers assist them in finding the right bras and prostheses. "They walk out the door smiling and confident with how they look," she says.

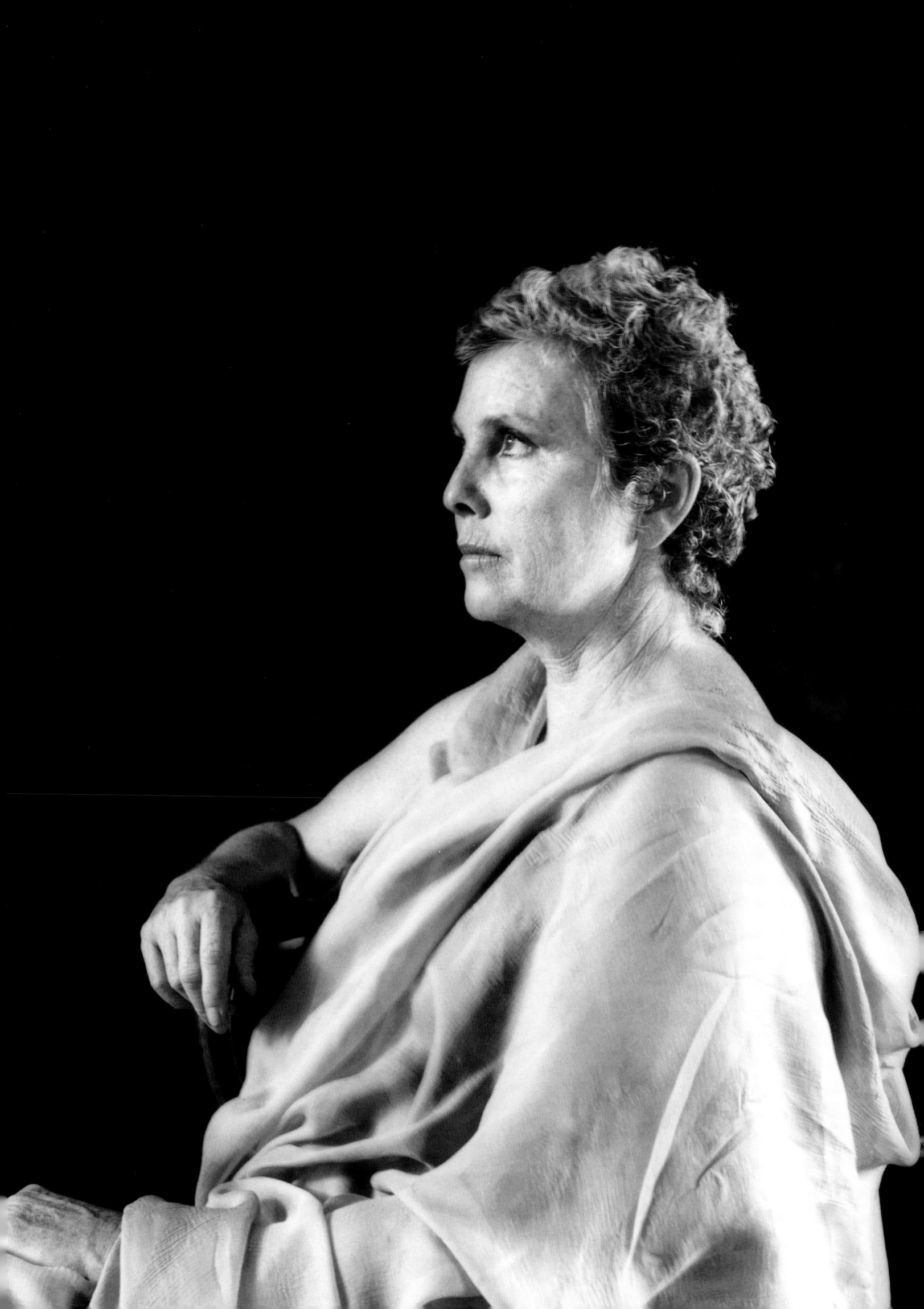

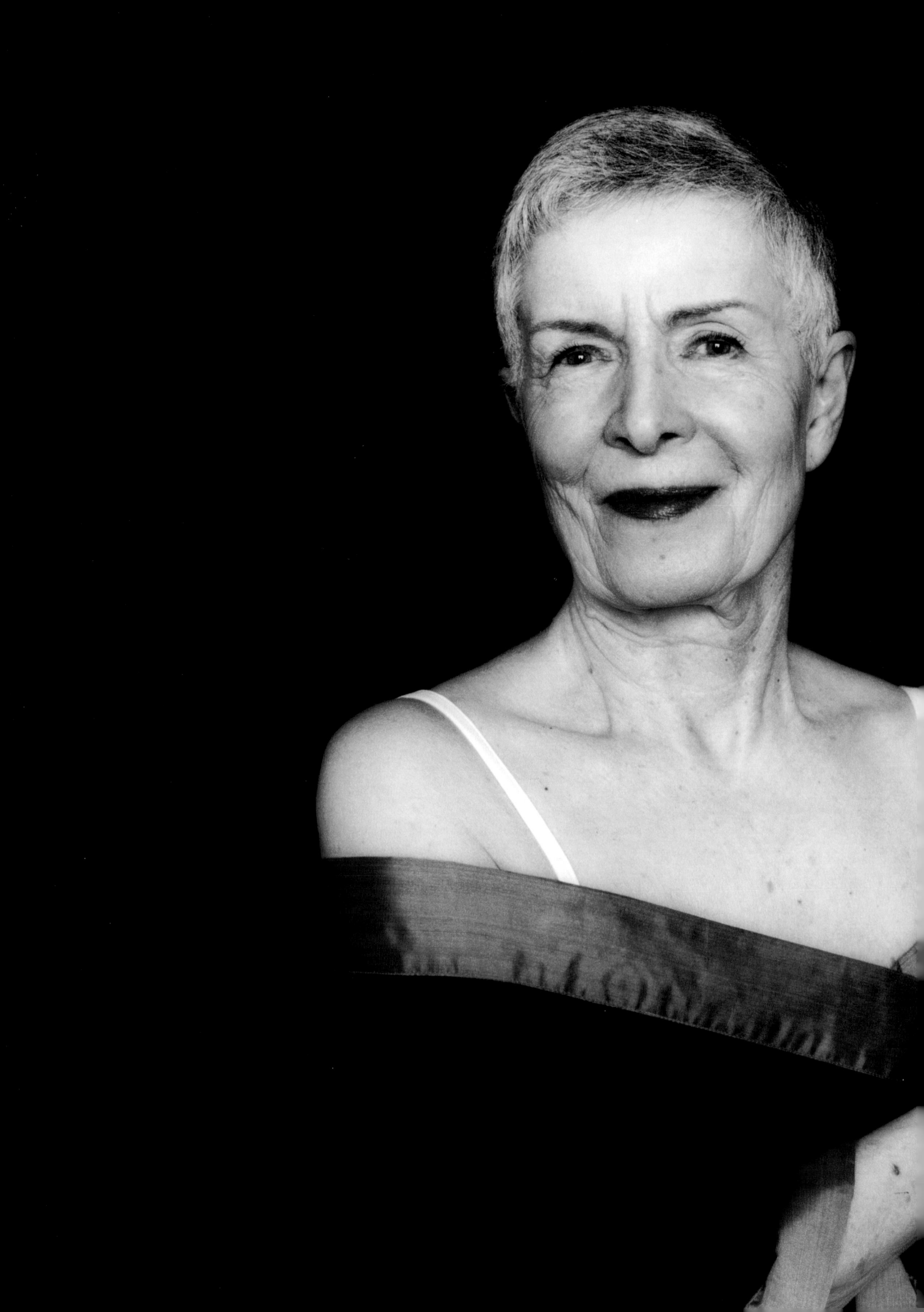

Lois

The challenges of breast cancer inspired Lois Tschetter Hjelmstad, who spent her pre-diagnosis days teaching piano and caring for her family, to venture into the world of publishing. Her greatest fear was of dying, and she found that writing brought her validation and comfort—two things she now brings to her readers, many of whom are dealing with similar issues. She has published two books, the latest of which is *The Last Violet: Mourning My Mother*. Her writings have opened up other opportunities for her, and Lois has traveled more than 200,000 miles from her Englewood, Colorado, home to share her message with women and those who care for them.

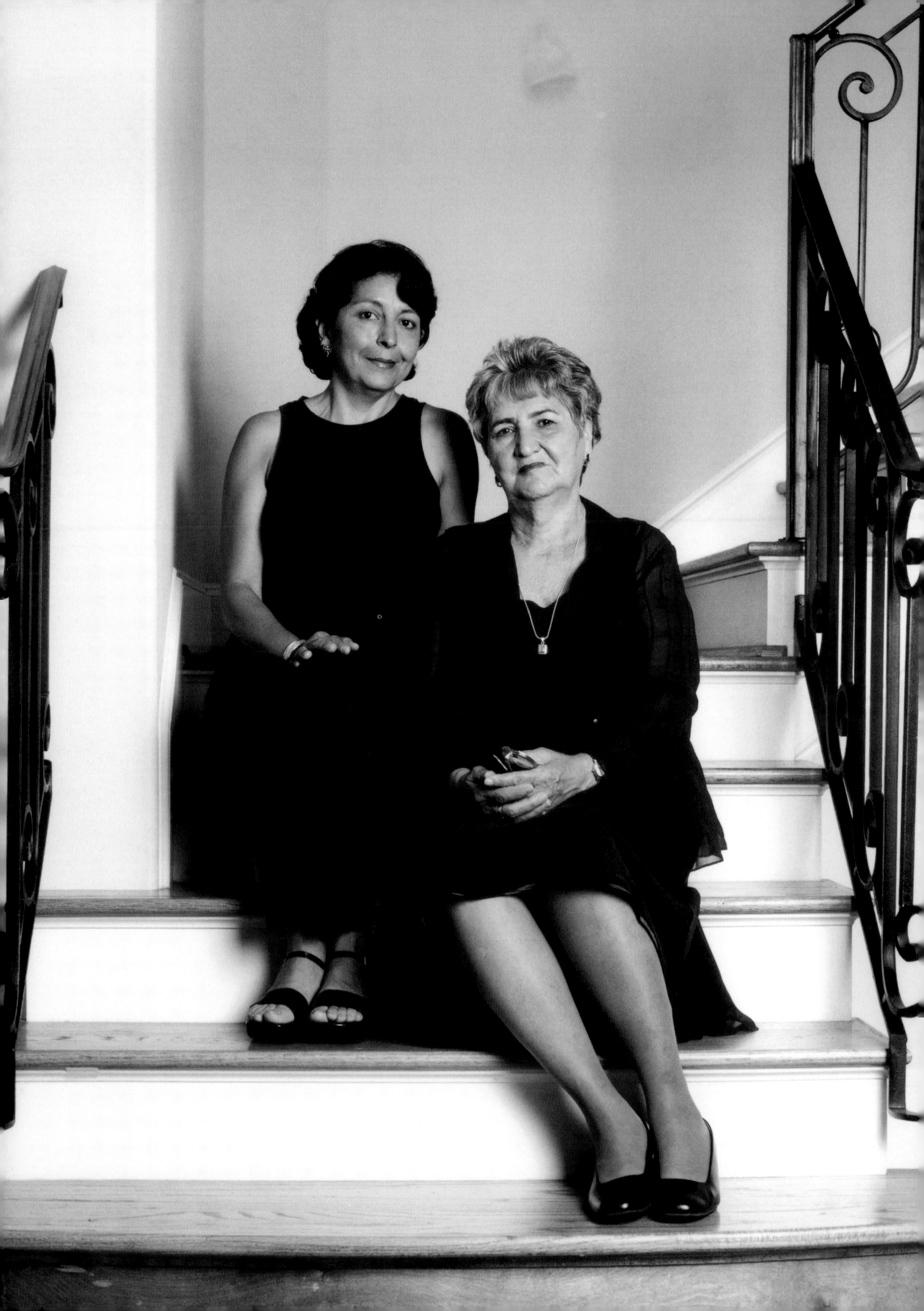

Lourdes and Eufracia

Lourdes Hernandez's mother, Eufracia, is her hero. Lourdes had two reoccurrences of breast cancer before her mother's diagnosis in 2001. Eufracia Hernandez dealt with the disease with grace, strength, and determination, and Lourdes says it was an honor to help her mother through her treatment. "My mother raised five children on minimum wage, moving us from Mexico to the Imperial Valley on the Mexican border," she says. "She always knew we would get through it."

Lourdes left the corporate world to focus on her own health and her family. Today she works with the Susan G. Komen Breast Cancer Foundation and with Houston's MD Anderson Cancer Center to educate Hispanic women about breast cancer. The demographic has a low incidence of breast cancer, but a high mortality rate resulting from a failure to be proactive in seeking treatment. "This is my calling," she says. "The corporate world can wait."

In her book *First You Cry*, Betty Rollin was one of the first women to deal publicly and honestly with breast cancer. "These days, I have a lot of company—other women who have been struck, who also keep waking up each morning," she says in the book's epilogue. "We're a grateful bunch. We know perfectly well we could have died—still could from a recurrence—yet we've been lucky. It's funny how lucky cancer makes you feel. Not at first, but later."

A New Yorker, Betty is an award-winning broadcast journalist who is a contributing correspondent for both NBC News and PBS. But she didn't discover her love for writing books until her experience with cancer motivated her to put pen to paper.

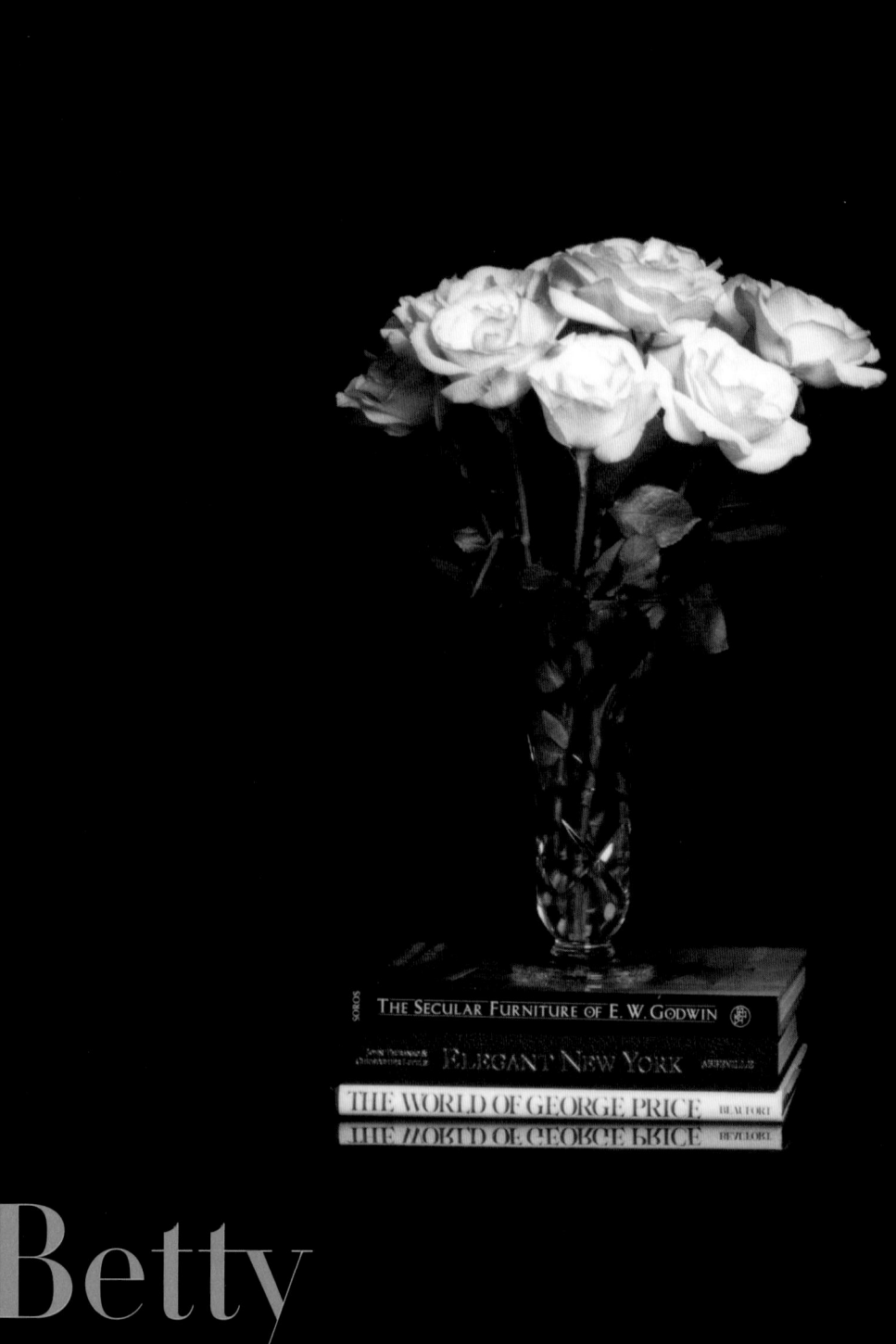

Betty

122

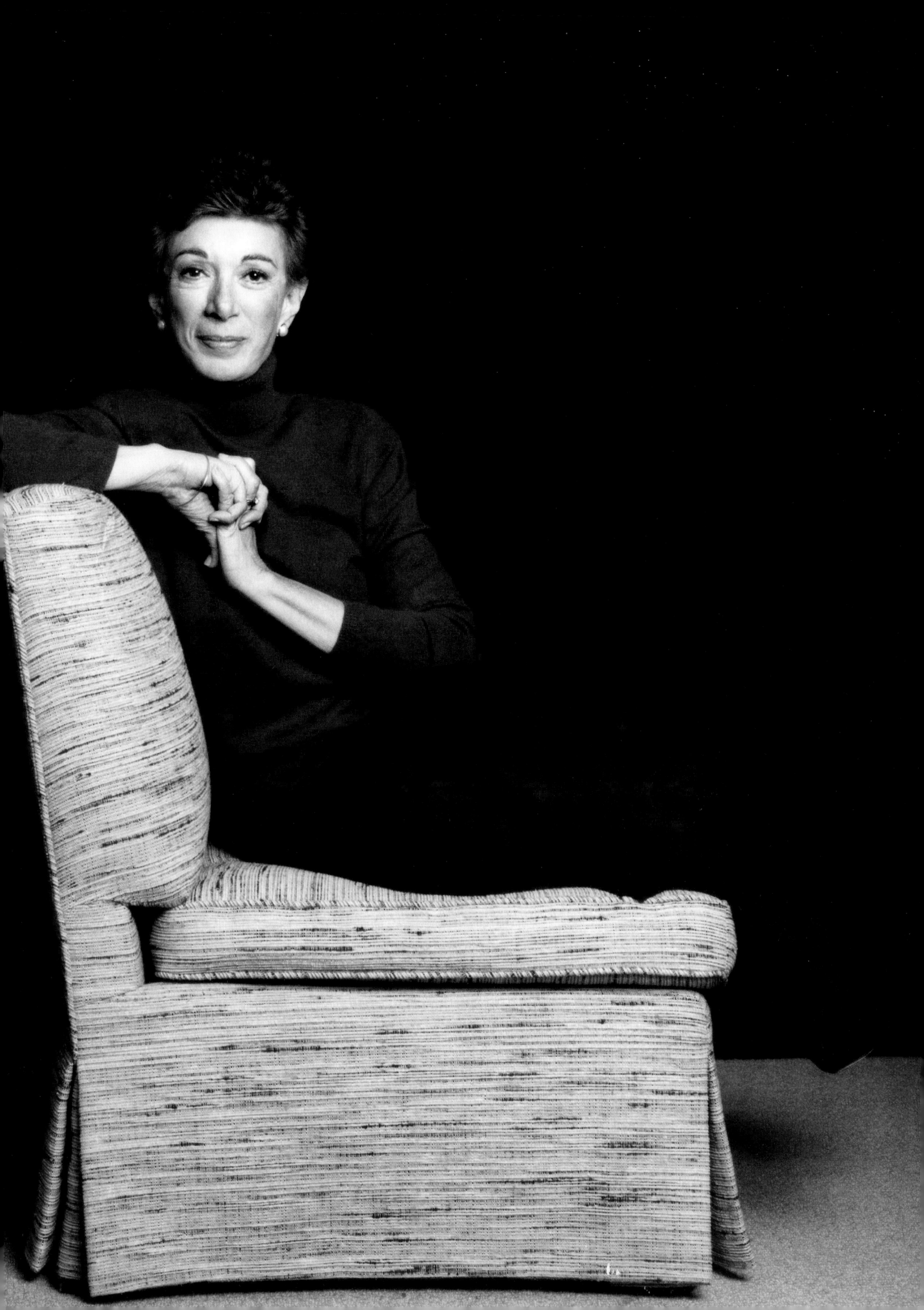

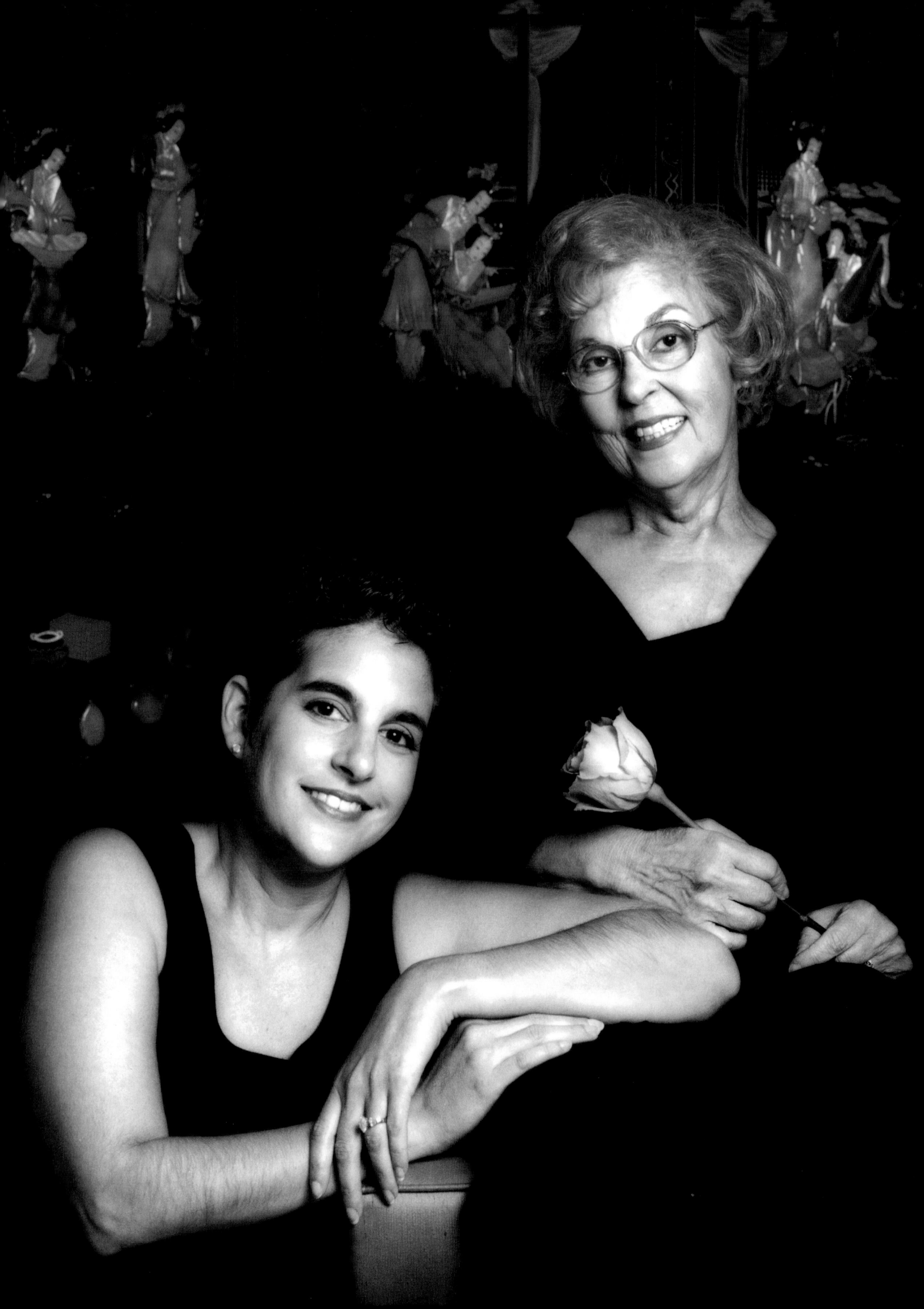

Marcia and Nell

Marcia Levine says her mother, Nell Prager, is "a perfect example of a true survivor." Nell—whose own mother, Rose (represented by the rose in the image here), had died of breast cancer—was diagnosed with the disease forty years ago at age forty, and underwent a double-mastectomy. Her strength would serve as a model for Marcia. A stay-at-home mom raising three daughters, Marcia was first diagnosed at age thirty-one, and then again at age thirty-four.

Pat

Patricia McKeever's mother and sister both lost their battles with breast cancer. So when Pat was diagnosed in 1990 at the age of forty-two, she was particularly frightened. At that time she was giving piano lessons and pursuing a master's degree in fine arts, all while staying at home to care for her four children. "I always believed in seizing the day, and I thought I was in control. Thought is an understatement," she says. "I decided I was going to beat this. I prayed hard, and I meditated every night in my bubble bath."

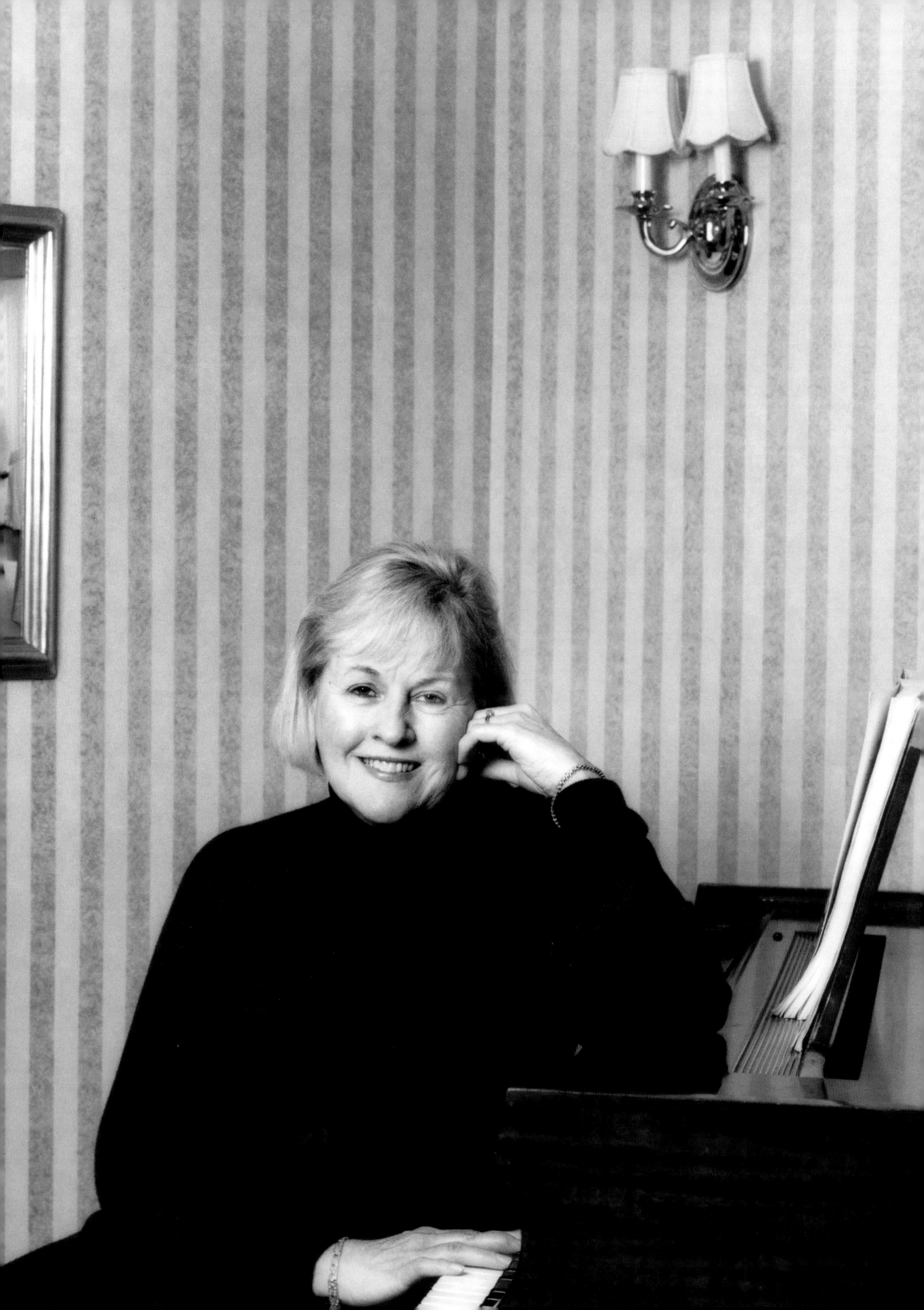

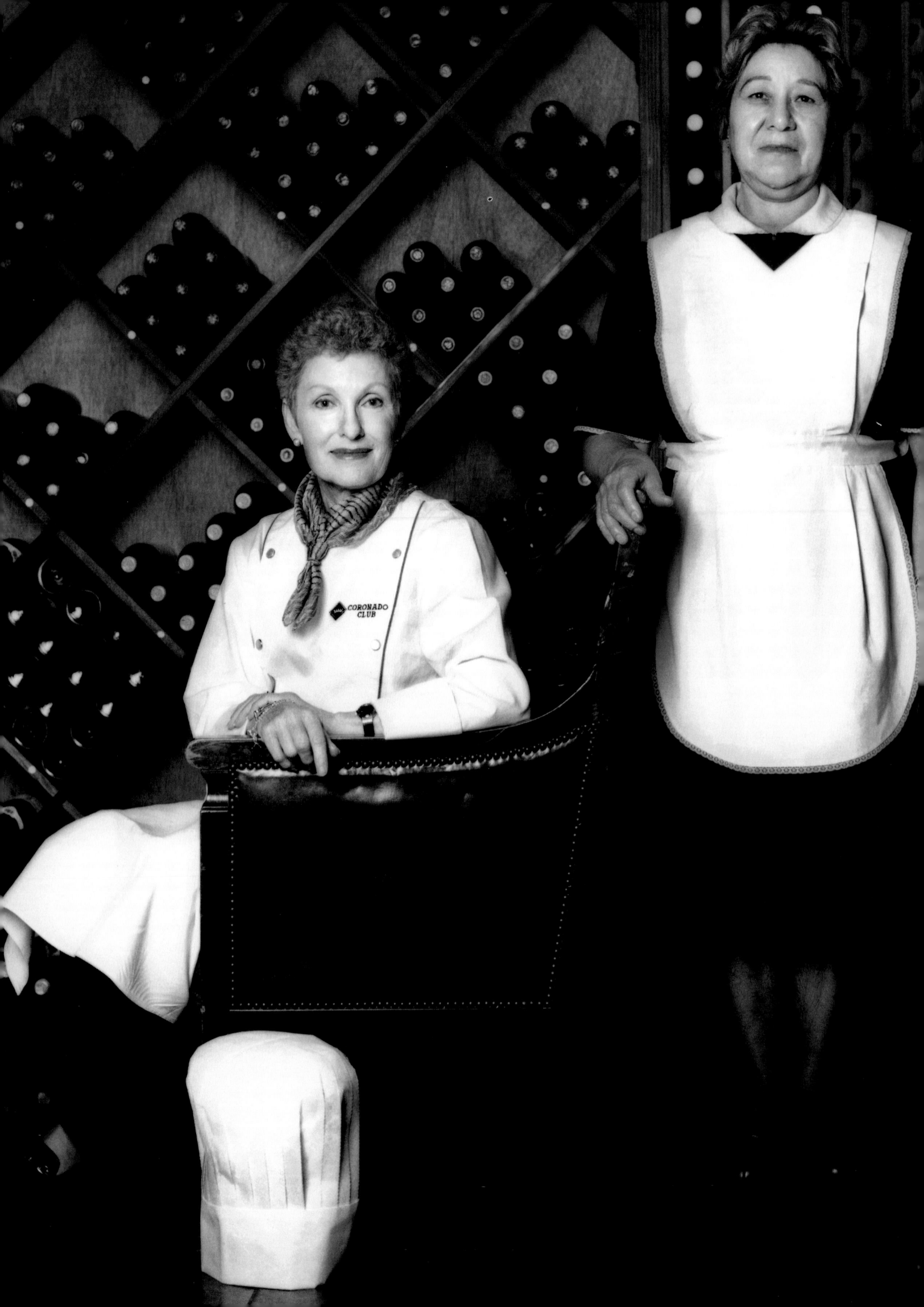

Mary Nell and Lucha

When Mary Nell Reck started cooking at the age of seven, she found her true calling—one that would lead to a twenty-eight-year career as a chef and restaurateur. After she was diagnosed with breast cancer at age fifty-six, she reached a defining moment in her life when she decided to surrender to the disease rather than fight it. From that point on, she devoted herself to traveling with her family to her farm in the south of France and spending time in her herb and vegetable garden. She is pictured here with Lucha Gutierrez, a coworker at the Coronado Club in Houston (where Mary Nell was the chef and manager) and fellow breast cancer survivor. *Mary Nell died in November 2003 at the age of sixty.*

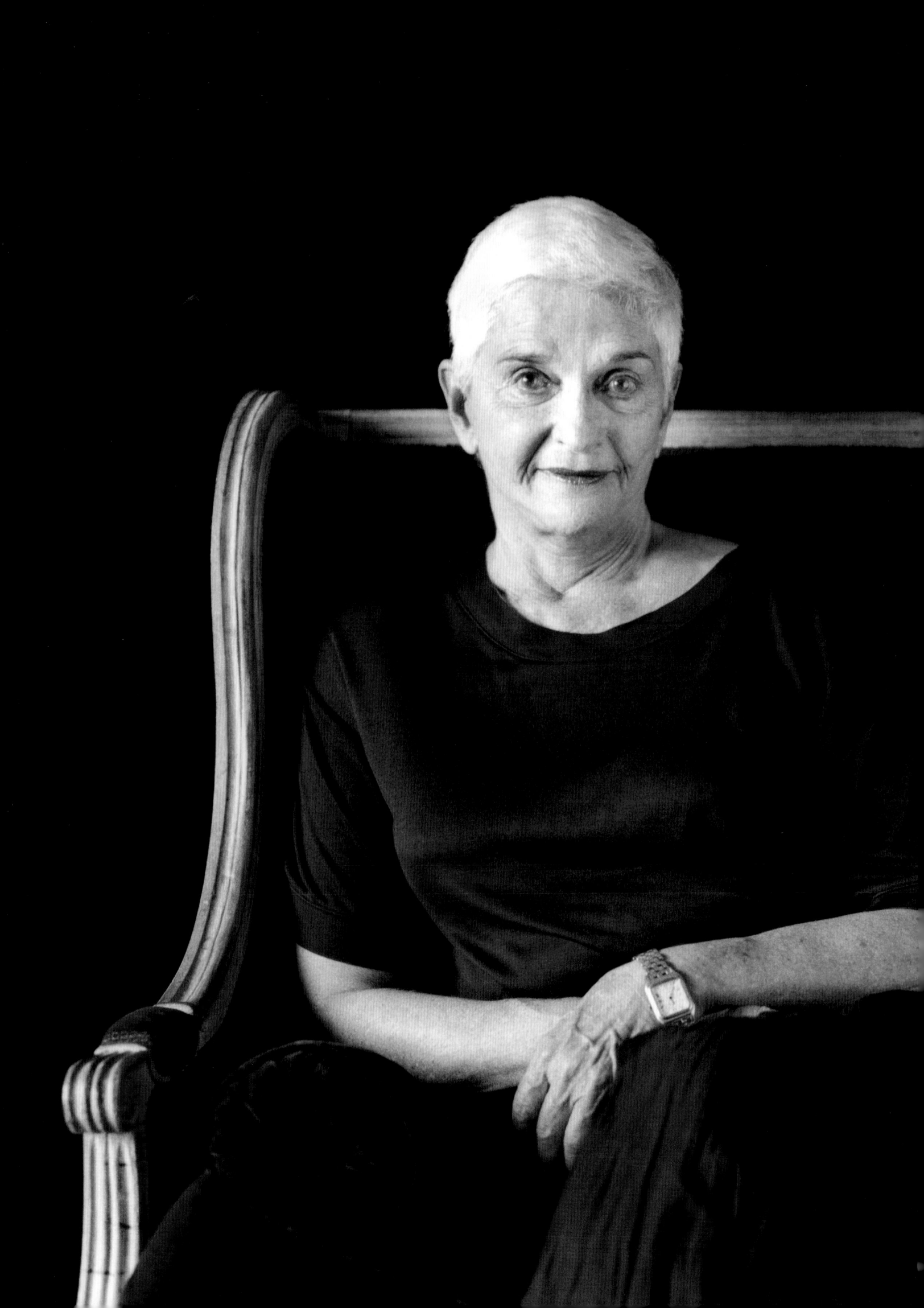

Sissy

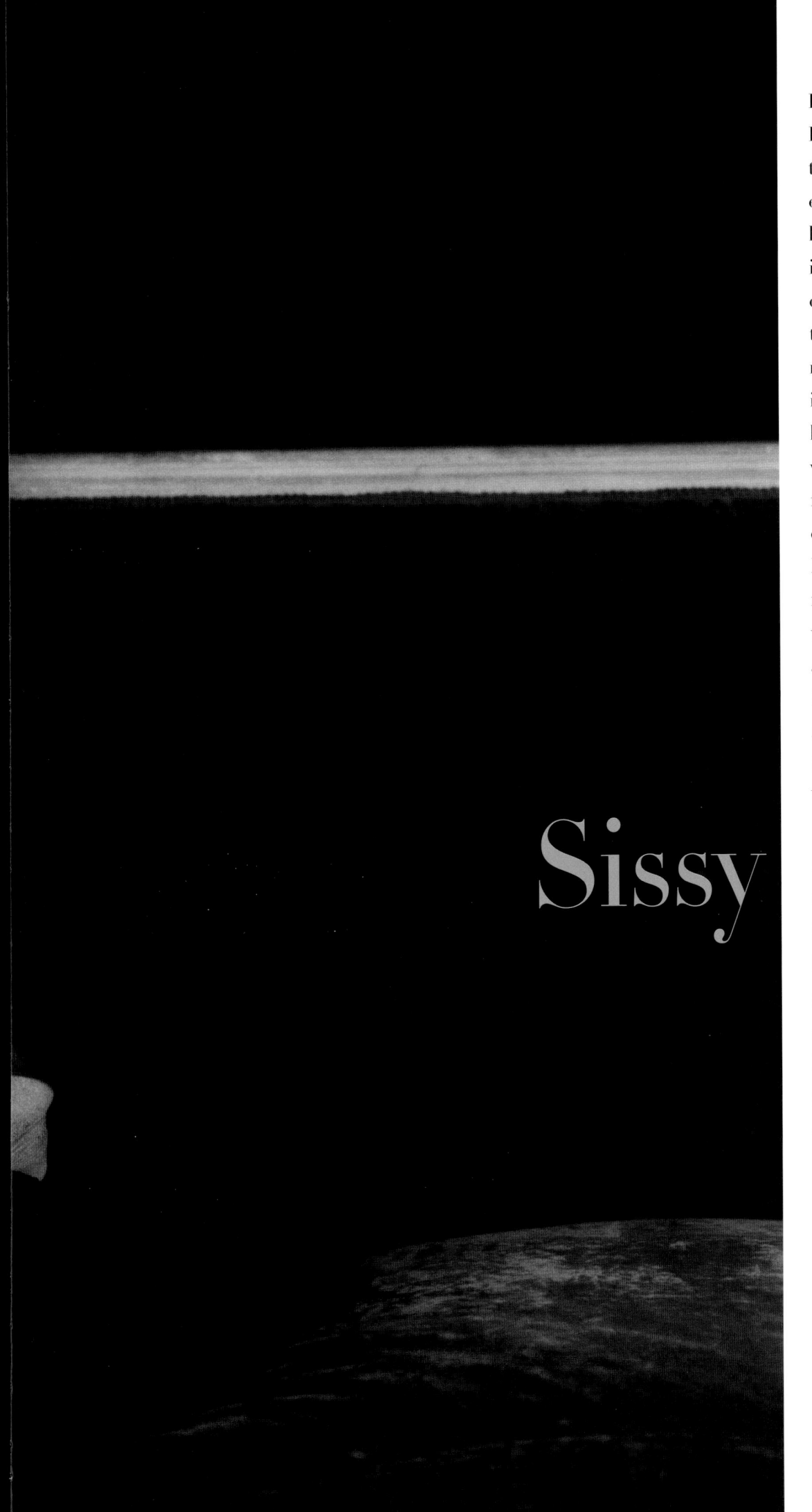

Frances "Sissy" Farenthold, who became the first woman to be elected to the Texas legislature in 1968, isn't intimidated when the odds are against her. By the time she was diagnosed with breast cancer in 1995, she had already been fighting for women's issues and for gender equity for decades through two Democratic gubernatorial campaigns, a vice-presidential nod at the 1972 Democratic National Convention, and her term as the first female president of Wells College.

A pioneer for women in the political arena and out, Sissy also has used her political platform to be a strong advocate for nationwide studies that explore the causes of breast cancer—an issue that hits close to home with this dynamic activist.

Jean and Florence

My mother, Florence Levy, and I have survived breast cancer's repeated visits to the women in our family. My mother has felt its impact the most strongly—she has seen her mother and sister both lose their battles with breast cancer, has suffered through her own diagnoses of first one breast and then the other, and has witnessed my own mastectomy and reconstruction. For this reason, I was moved to combine my portrayal of my mother's courage and strength with my own self-portrait photograph here.

"I was worried about it, naturally, and a little paranoid," she says about the first time she went to her doctor with a suspicious "dimple" on her breast. "I knew it was not good." But she waited until after my wedding to confirm her suspicions.

Once she knew she was fighting the same disease that had already claimed the lives of two of her loved ones, she says she tried to calm her fears by keeping busy. "I don't know what I did to stay so busy, but I stayed busy. The only time I thought about it was at night when I'd go to bed." She says she shared her fears during those dark nights with my father, Harry, who would always assure her she'd be fine. She admits that she didn't believe him, but she still found his words comforting.

Even today, with her mastectomies behind them and sixty-five years of marriage shared between them, my father still tells my mom that she's beautiful.

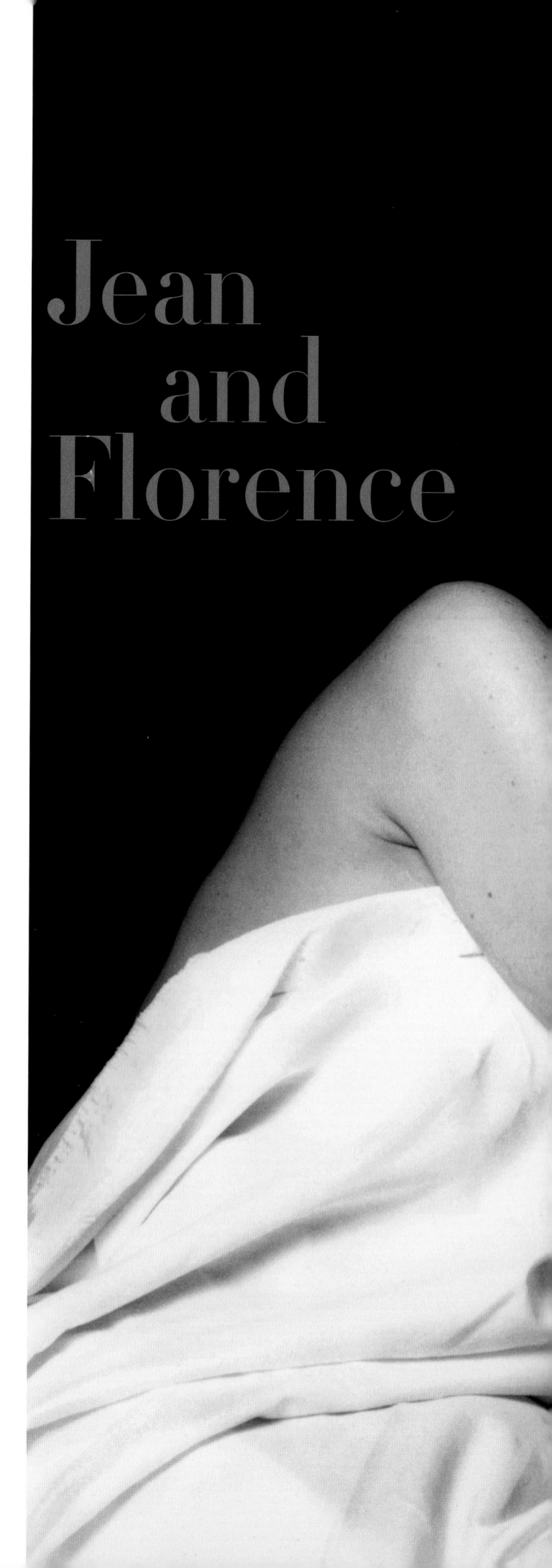

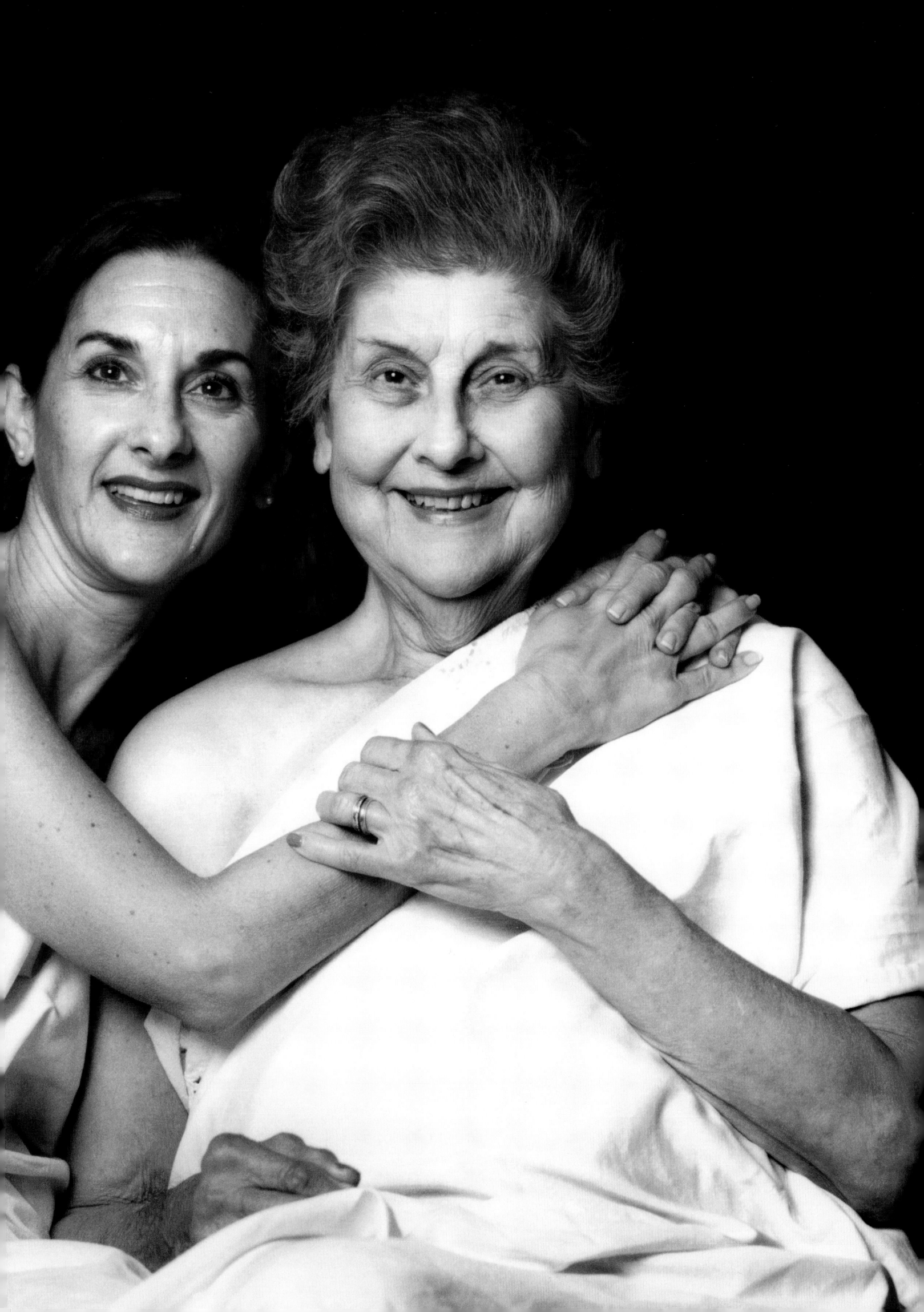

Resources

The following resources have been cited by the women featured within these pages. Contact your local chapter of the American Cancer Society or the Susan G. Komen Foundation for information about support available near you.

DanceLife Productions Inc.
Non-profit organization dedicated to promoting breast cancer awareness through the arts
445 W. 50th St., Suite 3E
New York, NY 10019
(212) 877-8441
www.dancelifenyc.org

Common Cares Foundation
Non-profit support group providing bilingual medical assistance, education, and counseling for cancer patients, spouses, families, and the indigent
11661 Preston Road #154
Dallas, TX 75230
(214) 365-9165
www.commoncares.org

Pink Ribbons Project
The first non-profit dance organization to promote awareness about breast cancer and to help raise funding for breast cancer advocacy, research, and education
1210 West Clay # 3
Houston, TX 77019
(713) 526-1907, ext.# 2
www.pinkribbons.org

Susan G. Komen Foundation
Working through a network of U.S. and international affiliates and hosting events like the Race for the Cure, the Komen Foundation is fighting to eradicate breast cancer as a life-threatening disease by funding research grants and supporting education, screening, and treatment projects in communities around the world.
5005 LBJ Freeway, Suite 250
Dallas, TX 75244
(972) 855-1600
Helpline: 1-800-I'M AWARE
www.komen.org

SHARE
A non-profit organization that offers peer-led support to women with breast or ovarian cancer, as well as to their families and friends
1501 Broadway #1720
New York, NY 10036
(212) 719-0364
Toll-free 1-866-891-2392
www.sharecancer
support.org

American Cancer Society
Chinese Support Units
Flushing, New York:
(718) 886-8890
Fords, New Jersey:
(732) 225-8588
Parsippany, New Jersey:
(973) 334-2249
Shrewsbury, New Jersey:
(732) 224-8868
Northern California:
(510) 797-0600

Women of Faith and Hope
A religiously oriented self-help group for African-American women in the Philadelphia region to support and educate them before, during, and after breast cancer diagnosis and treatment
Contact Novella Lyons at
(215) 985-5303

Harley's Angels Calendar
Proceeds from sales of the Harley's Angels Calendar are donated for cancer research.
Contact Kimen Metzger at
(713) 896-4502
www.cruzintocure.com

Photographs

Jerri Nielsen
PAGE 2

Carolyn Farb
PAGE 4

Leah Garmon
PAGE 6

Martha Carrillo
PAGE 8

Susan Rafte
PAGE 10

Dana Ravel
PAGE 12

Monica Yaniv
PAGE 14

Donna Dohmann and
Carrie Wood
PAGE 16

Carol Horn
PAGE 18

Marcy Langer
PAGE 20

Liz Riedel
PAGE 22

Pam Vaughn
PAGE 24

J.B. Pena
PAGE 26

Angela and David Weber
PAGE 28

Oni Faida Lampley
PAGE 30

Susan Massin
PAGE 32

Liz Carpenter
PAGE 34

Joy Luck Club
PAGE 36 AND 38

Marty Leonard
PAGE 40

Phoebe Wood
PAGE 42

Mary Walsh
PAGE 44

Pearle Griffith-Eccles
PAGE 46

Gayle Clark
PAGE 48

Laura Miller
PAGE 50

Elizabeth Merritt
PAGE 52

Jane E. Pollock
PAGE 54

Bitsy Proler
PAGE 56

Lyudmila
Rudyakov
PAGE 58

Ann Hudson and
Eugenia Lara
PAGE 60

Dr. Alan Johns
PAGE 62

Peggy Perry
PAGE 64

Christine Nix
PAGE 66

Lois, Shakay, Gloria,
Pearl, Elena, Lisa
PAGE 68

Darrell Kirkland
PAGE 70

Fran Shelton
PAGE 72

Julie Ann Janaszak
and Judith Ann Olson
PAGE 74

Joan Katz
PAGE 76

Elaine Saltsman
PAGE 78

Dottie Montoya
PAGE 80

Lisa Conwell
PAGE 82

Gloria Stuart
PAGE 84

Elyse Clark
PAGE 86

Barbara Flood
PAGE 88

Laura Beattie
PAGE 90

Harley's Angels
PAGE 92

Lois Chiles
PAGE 94

Susan Gillette
PAGE 96

Leslie Mouton Mattox
PAGE 98

Novella Lyons
PAGE 100

Elfriede Gerland
PAGE 102

Valentina Markusova
PAGE 104

Karen McCulley
PAGE 106

Jill
PAGE 108

Cynthia Hudson
PAGE 110

Laurie Jensen
PAGE 112

Karen Faulkner Key
PAGE 114

Jana Johnson
PAGE 116

Lois Tschetter
Hjelmstad
PAGE 118

Lourdes and
Eufracia Hernandez
PAGE 120

Betty Rollin
PAGE 122

Marcia Levine and
Nell Prager
PAGE 124

Patricia McKeever
PAGE 126

Mary Nell Reck
and Lucha Gutierrez
PAGE 128

Frances "Sissy"
Farenthold
PAGE 130

Jean Karotkin and
Florence Levy
PAGE 132

About the Author

Jean Karotkin is a Dallas-based photographer whose work has been featured in national magazines including *O, The Oprah Magazine* and *Rosie Magazine*, as well as on NBC's *Today* show. Her photographs were part of an exhibition at the Houston Center for Photography, and have been widely exhibited at other venues to benefit and raise awareness of breast cancer. *Body & Soul* is the first collection of her photography in book form.